Jeannette Ewin Ph.D. is a r
with an international follow   ...pleted her
doctorate in human anatomy and biochemistry, and
received a Fellowship in the Department of Nutrition at
the Harvard University School of Public Health. After years
in scientific research and health care administration, her
interest in preventative medicine drew her back to the
field of nutrition. Community education on food and
health is now her primary interest.

'New Perspectives' series

'New Perspectives' provide attractive and accessible introductions to a comprehensive range of mind, body, and spirit topics. Beautifully designed and illustrated, these practical books are written by experts in each subject.

Books in the series:

Alexander Technique, Richard Brennan
Crystal Therapy, Stephanie and Tim Harrison
Homeopathy, Peter Adams
Nutritional Therapy, Jeannette Ewin

New Perspectives

NUTRITIONAL THERAPY

An Introductory Guide to the Healing Power of Food

JEANETTE EWIN

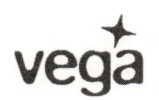

vega

© Vega 2002
Text © Jeannette Ewin 2000, 2002

All rights reserved. No part of this book may be reproduced, stored in a retrieval system or transmitted in any form or by any means, electronic, mechanical, photocopying, recording or otherwise, without the prior permission in writing of the copyright owners

ISBN 1-84333-519-0

A catalogue record for this book is available from the British Library

First published in 2002 by
Vega
64 Brewery Road
London, N7 9NT

A member of **Chrysalis** Books plc

Visit our website at www.chrysalisbooks.co.uk

Printed in Great Britain
by CPD, Wales

Contents

1 Healing with Food 7

2 Nutritional Therapy and You 17

3 How Nutritional Therapy Works 25

4 Digestion: Turning Food into Molecules 40

5 What Food Contains 47

6 Miracles From Plants 65

7 Food Supplements 74

8 Self-help and Disease Prevention 83

9 Food and Beauty 104

10 Consulting a Nutritional Therapist 108

11 Taking it Further 113

Glossary 116

Further Reading 119

Useful Addresses 121

Index 125

Acknowledgements

No author is productive without help from others. Among those I wish to thank for their contributions to this book are the people at Design Revolution, and in particular Nicola Hodgson.

The nutritional therapist, Antony Haynes, also deserves my heartfelt thanks for applying his skills, extensive knowledge and humanity to my personal illness. It is to him, and to all others who drive forward the science and application of nutrition to human illness, that this book is dedicated.

Note from the Publisher
Any information given in any book in the New Perspectives series is not intended to be taken as a replacement for medical advice. Any person with a condition requiring medical attention should consult a qualified medical practitioner or suitable therapist.

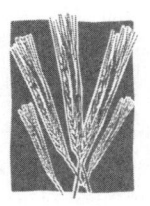

HEALING WITH FOOD

CHAPTER ONE

Why should anyone read a book about nutritional therapy? Because food contains the power of life. The food and drink that we choose to consume can have a profound effect on our health and well-being. Nutrition is the intimate link between ourselves and the rest of the living world. Everything we need for health can be found in the edible plants and animals around us. In a healthy person, a delicate harmony, or balance, exists between the nutrients the body needs and the nutrients received from the diet. When this balance is disrupted – by accidents, infection, or poor food choices – well-being is threatened and illness may result. Nutritional therapy seeks to identify imbalance and restore health through food.

Using food to restore and maintain health is not a new idea. Modern nutritional therapy has its roots in ancient traditions, such as the Indian Ayurvedic system and traditional Chinese medicine. Recent scientific findings often bear out the folk knowledge of ancient healing systems. For example, the earliest writings considered part of the heritage of modern medicine appeared in the Kahun and

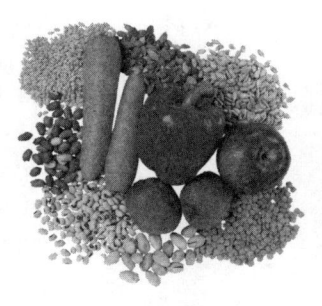

ABOVE MANY SYSTEMS OF HEALING MAINTAIN THAT EATING A WELL-BALANCED DIET IS FUNDAMENTAL TO GOOD HEALTH.

Ebers papyri, written about 3,500 years ago. These papyri included the observation that eating liver was a good treatment for night blindness. Scientists now know that the liver stores vitamin A, and that vitamin A is essential for night vision.

AYURVEDIC HEALING

The foundations of Ayurveda developed from ancient Hindu scriptures (Vedas) written 3,500–4000 years ago. It is said that fifty-two wise and holy men of India journeyed to the foothills of the Himalayas in search of ways to eliminate disease from the world. Through meditation, they received divine inspiration, which they recorded and began to practise.

Ayurveda is a holistic system of healing based on the idea of harmony between people and their environment. These ideas are increasingly appealing to people in the modern Western world. According to Ayurvedic belief, we and everything else in the universe are made up of five elements that should be held in balance. There are also thought to be three vital energies, or doshas, in the body that should be kept in harmony. The three doshas are vata, pitta and kapha. Kapha is water and earth, pitta is fire and water, and vata is ether and air. Each dosha influences specific parts of the body: for example, pitta most affects the digestive system, excluding the small and large intestines, which are influenced by vata. Kapha influences the respiratory system.

The doshas also reflect the Western idea of body types. Kapha people are heavy-framed and associated with the colour yellow; pitta people are of medium build and associated

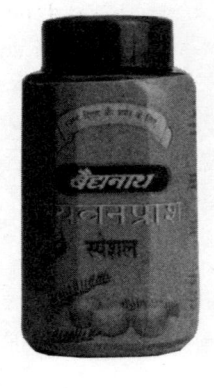

LEFT THE ANCIENT INDIAN SYSTEM OF HEALING KNOWN AS AYURVEDA EMPHASISES THE IMPORTANCE OF BALANCE AND HARMONY.

with red; and lean and delicate people are vata, identified by the colour blue. Each of us is a combination of the doshas, although one usually predominates.

The knowledge used in modern Ayurveda builds on its ancient teaching and knowledge from philosophy, astrology, psychology and astronomy. It also borrows from modern medical teaching and modern nutrition. The belief that the mind and the body must be understood and treated as one is central to Ayurveda, and meditation and yoga are often used to control stress and stress-related illness. In conjunction with this, the body is treated through diet, herbal remedies, massage and cleansing practices. Among the basic dietary rules of Ayurveda are:

- Food should be a source of pleasure and nourishment.
- Food should be of the best quality, served at a moderate temperature, consumed at a modest pace and enjoyed in a clean and pleasant environment.
- Talking and laughing during meals should be avoided, as this causes movements in the stomach that slow digestion.
- Ingredients should be as close to 'natural' as possible.
- Foods are assigned seasons in which they are best purchased and eaten. Sweet food should be avoided in the spring, as the body is slow to burn off calories. In summer, sweet, cold foods cool the body. In winter, comforting, warm foods can be enjoyed, such as honey, milk, rice and oil.

There are interesting crossovers between Ayurvedic practice and the growing body of modern scientific information about healing compounds in foods. Many of the spices used in Ayurvedic cookery are now known to contain healing properties. For example, scientists are currently exploring the anticancer, anti-inflammatory and antioxidant powers of curcumin, a compound found in turmeric.

RIGHT TURMERIC, A SPICE COMMONLY USED IN AYURVEDIC COOKERY, MAY CONTAIN CANCER-FIGHTING COMPOUNDS.

Traditional Chinese Medicine

The complex theoretical foundations of Traditional Chinese medicine are based on millennia of close observation. Illnesses are diagnosed through observation, structured interviews, palpation of the pulse in various parts of the body, and diagnostic acupuncture. Besides the prescription of dietary change and healing herbs, treatment takes the form of massage, acupuncture and moxibustion (a means of treating pain in which a cone of woodworm leaves [moxa] is burned just above the skin).

In Chinese philosophy, all things consist of two counter-forces; for example, inside and outside; heat and cold; expansion and contraction; excess and deficiency. This duality within wholeness, known as Yin/Yang, is a basic concept that also influences Chinese diet therapy. For good health and harmony within the body, yin and yang must be balanced. Therefore, if an illness produces the perception of heat, it should be treated with a cooling food. In contrast, a condition causing a patient to feel cold should be treated with a food producing heat. People suffering from a toxic condition require detoxifying foods, and those suffering from deficiency are treated with 'building' foods. A person with excessive yang, which might manifest itself as a high fever, needs to be treated with yin foods such as millet, barley, beets and watermelon.

Traditional Chinese medicine began to be known in the West in the early 1970s, when the 'Barefoot Doctors', who met most of the medical needs of the country, prepared a medical manual describing the methods that they used. The Barefoot Doctors were peasant farmers and other rural inhabitants who were trained as para-medics to introduce basic public health changes and provide primary care services. They used a combination of acupuncture, interview

LEFT MAINTAINING BALANCE BETWEEN THE OPPOSING FORCES OF YIN AND YANG IS A FUNDAMENTAL CONCEPT OF TRADITIONAL CHINESE MEDICINE.

techniques, modernized herbal treatment, and various aspects of Western medical knowledge. The publication of the manual was an effort to preserve part of a history that had served China well, so that it could be integrated with modern medical teaching into a system of treatment that best suited the people of that nation. The manual was subsequently translated and published in the United States and Great Britain, with an appendix summarising scientific evidence suggesting the medical effectiveness of 45 plants and herbal preparations used by the Barefoot Doctors. More remedies and healing techniques have since been shown to exhibit medical value.

Barefoot Doctors gradually lost their importance as Western medicine was more widely accepted in China. However, the Western world is taking an increased interest in traditional Chinese medicine.

HIPPOCRATES

Hippocrates (460–377 BC) – the Greek father of modern medicine – recommended many herbal concoctions and manipulations of the diet in his major work on medical treatments, *Regimens*.
For example, he suggested that eating liver is good for the eyes (and liver contains vitamin A, which prevents night blindness) and suggested that honey is a healing food (it does in fact have antibacterial properties). He also suggested that starchy foods are most difficult to digest in the summer and autumn, and easiest in winter.

Hippocrates recognised that we are an intimate part of the world around us. In another of his most important works, *Airs, Waters, Places*, Hippocrates suggested a connection between environment and disease, and environment and cure. It seems that during the two millennia since Hippocrates' death we have done little more than further investigate the nature of disease, and rediscover the validity of his basic concepts of health.

Nutrition in the Modern Age

Several ancient systems of medicine emphasised the link between balance in nutrition and good health. However, European cultures have had a more haphazard history in determining how nutritional deficiencies can cause illness. The curse of both modern medicine and the science of nutrition is to discover and rediscover, and still fail to apply what has been learned. The history of scurvy is a case in point. Scurvy is a terrible disease caused by a deficiency in vitamin C that leads to both madness and deadly bleeding. Scurvy curtailed the empire-building of the ancient Romans when their troops in the colder parts of Europe succumbed to the disease, for which they had no cure.

Several observers over the years recorded potential cures for scurvy, but their knowledge was never acted upon. For example, the great French navigator Jacques Cartier in 1535 travelled with three ships to Canada. The ships became icebound in the St. Lawrence River. Food ran short, and most of the crew developed scurvy. After five months, one man, although ill himself, left the ship to find help. He returned completely recovered. A group of Indians that he encountered told him to eat 'leaves of the white cedar' (pine needles), which cured him. We now know that pine needles contain vitamin C, as well as other antioxidants.

In 1601, when the Dutch East India Company was first trading in the Far East, sailors fell ill with scurvy on all the vessels in the fleet but one. The ship was captained by Sir James Lancaster, whose ship's rations included lemons. This was reported in 1617, when the Dutch East Company's medical officer wrote, 'the use of the juice of lemon is a precious medicine and well tried ... Let it have chief place in the cure of the scurvy for it will deserve it...' These wise words went largely unheeded.

Evidence of the first controlled scientific study showing the effect of a specific food on the development of disease also involved scurvy. A naval surgeon, James Lind, recorded in 1753 how patients treated with two oranges and a lemon each day survived the ravages of scurvy, while those given cider, vinegar or a tincture of sulphuric acid did not. Lind's work made a greater impact on medical thinking of the time than Cartier's because he reported an objective 'experiment', in which he had demonstrated the positive effect of one food over others. Sadly, it took many years before this knowledge was used by the Royal Navy to protect its sailors from disease.

RIGHT WESTERN MEDICINE TOOK CENTURIES TO ACT ON THE KNOWLEDGE THAT VITAMIN C COULD PREVENT SCURVY.

Accidental Discovery

The substance in lemons responsible for their seemingly miraculous power to cure scurvy, vitamin C, was not discovered until the disease could be studied under laboratory conditions. The man who finally isolated the vitamin, as ascorbic acid, was Albert Szent-Gyorgi. He received the Nobel Prize for Medicine for his work in 1937. It is claimed that Szent-Gyorgi had trouble finding a rich source of what he knew would be the vitamin he sought. One night his wife prepared a meal that he found foul-tasting and inedible. While his wife was not looking, the scientist threw most of his dinner away, but saved a little, as the offensive taste seemed somehow familiar. Szent-Gyorgi took it to his laboratory, where he found that the dish was high in ascorbic acid. His wife had prepared Hungarian goulash, and had been heavy-handed with the paprika – a red pepper – which provided so much ascorbic acid that Szent-Gyorgi could produce from it the pure crystals he needed for his research.

Exploring the Link Between Food and Disease

It was not until the 19th century that the systematic experimentation on the relationship between food and disease began in earnest. Technology advanced to the point where the constituents of food could be separated and studied. The macronutrients (see pp.49–53) were explored first: protein, carbohydrates, fats. Next came the micronutrients: minerals and vitamins. Scientists began to identify many of the substances that are now known to be essential for human

The Controversy of RDAs

The scientific goal of establishing RDAs was admirable, and there are still many people today who feel they would benefit from knowing exactly how much of each nutrient they need. However, nutrition is not so simple and clear-cut, and RDAs have attracted controversy for this reason. RDAs reflected the needs of an average, healthy, young adult. They do not reflect the fact that nutritional requirements are influenced by age, sex, employment, activity level and health status, and whether the person smokes, takes recreational drugs or prescribed medicines. An individual's nutritional needs also change throughout life. Nutritional therapists recognise the unique physical needs and lifestyle demands of an individual, and frequently use specific nutrients in quantities far above those prescribed by RDAs.

New means of quantifying recommendations for essential nutrients have been developed, but for political reasons they have enjoyed little international agreement. For example, dietary recommendations for specific vitamins in America are not the same as those for Europeans, although, of course, human physiology is the same on both sides of the Atlantic Ocean.

health. Many researchers were surprised when they discovered that humans had different nutritional requirements from, for example, a goat or a chicken.

Once a substance was identified – be it a mineral, a vitamin, or a type of fat – its chemical characteristics were analysed. Attempts were then made to define exactly how much of the substance was needed for normal human health. The scientists' goal was to define the content of the ideal diet and establish the daily requirements of each essential nutrient. This led to the publication of RDAs (Recommended Daily Allowances – also known as Recommended Daily Amounts).

Research into nutrition began to stall at around the time of the Second World War. Scientists generally agreed that they had discovered just about all there was to know about human dietary requirements; more important were the emerging subjects of biochemistry and molecular biology. A subject that once fired popular imagination - and was dignified with awards of the Nobel Prize - fell from its place of importance among members of the medical community. Only recently has nutrition begun to regain scientific stature and interest.

THE FUTURE OF NUTRITIONAL DISCOVERIES

Today, interest in nutrition flourishes again in university research laboratories around the globe. In part inspired by the availability of advanced technology, scientists are at last truly seeking to understand the complex relationship between an individual's health and the food that she or he eats. Not afraid to seek answers from other sources of knowledge, many research nutritionists study herbal medicine, Ayurveda, traditional Chinese medicine, and other forms of healing. The answers that they are finding are exciting and hold real promise for a longer and healthier future for us all.

There are several large areas of research currently being explored, including:
- How nutrients interact with each other.
- The interaction between identified nutrients and other healing substances in plants.
- The identification of the very earliest signs of poor nutrition (or malnutrition), which occur long before serious changes, such as skin eruptions and psychotic episodes, are observable.
- The healing effects of doses of vitamins and minerals that are larger than those identified as adequate for the average human body.
- The interactions between the environment, an individual's lifestyle and his or her need for specific nutrients.

These are the challenges to modern nutritionists, and although they are far better equipped for this research, they have much to overcome both in bias and understanding of the complexities of human biology.

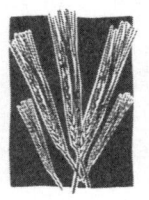

NUTRITIONAL THERAPY AND YOU

CHAPTER TWO

You are probably reading this book because you want to enjoy a long and active life. You may also want to improve your appearance. Is either possible? If you are like most of us, you already have one or two physical problems that concern you, and you are probably not on the list of the top ten international fashion models. However, you are who you are. You have your own unique and miraculous body to enjoy throughout your life.

To achieve the stamina and the vitality that are fundamental to a long and active life, you must learn to protect, enhance and maintain the substances and biological processes that make up your body. A balanced diet is the answer. You can look better, feel better and add years to a life of activity and enjoyment by knowing which foods to choose and enjoy at different stages of your life. It is highly unlikely that you can alter your external appearance to meet some media image of perfection. You can, however, realize maximum strength, energy and mental acuity. Life is to be enjoyed, and good nutrition is the foundation of life. (Exercise plays a vital part in maximizing your physical and mental potential, but your body must be properly nourished before it can take full advantage of sensible exercise.)

Throughout your life, proper nutrition will help you achieve a maximum state of 'well-being': a state of maximum physical and mental strength and stamina for your age, sex, lifestyle and state of health. That is something that is worth striving for.

'Perfect' Health and Well-being

I believe that the idea of 'health' has been corrupted by the media to mean 'perfect' health. That would involve every biological system in the body working perfectly and in balance all the time, even in the face of infection, stress and environmental pollution.

From reading stories in the popular press, it might seem possible that everyone can enjoy perfect health at all times. All we need do is change various dietary habits, or alter our living environment, and all our physical cares will disappear. We will be young and slim and free of illness. Real life does not work that way. Many diseases in Western society have complex causes that relate as much to the processes of ageing in the body as to external influences. We can significantly lower our risk of developing these diseases, but we will never be able to irradicate them, as science has done with infectious illnesses such as polio and smallpox.

What image comes to mind when you think of a person in perfect health? A happy young woman, slim, with swimsuit proportions and a family of three lively children? A young man with well-developed muscles and a good haircut: an athlete, perhaps, at the top of the podium during an Olympic Awards ceremony? Or, do you think of an 80-year-old woman walking briskly from the train towards her car after a day of business meetings. Or a 75-year-old man lifting foul-weather gear into his boat before he and his wife set sail on a fortnight's trip down the European coast? If you are like most people, the images of youth and beauty probably came to mind first. Yet youth alone does not ensure health.

None of these people may have an obvious illness, but it is possible that each suffers from at least one physical complaint. We know that some top athletes suffer from disorders as serious as diabetes. Many young women are affected by monthly bouts of pre-menstrual syndrome, or the feelings of tiredness associated with mild anaemia caused by iron deficiency. Many elderly people suffer to some degree from at least one degenerative illness, such as arthritis or high blood pressure. And any of this imagined group could have fought a battle with cancer and won. In other words, none enjoys 'perfect' health, but they all enjoy well-being.

When I consulted my doctor some years ago about a painful arthritic joint he said, 'get used to it, we all have to have something'. He was right, of course. As we grow older we all gradually develop problems. Some of them will be minor: constipation, indigestion or minor bouts of fatigue. (These can be helped through nutritional therapy, as you will see in a later chapter.) But some conditions that we may develop are very serious: diabetes, irritable bowel syndrome, a heart condition or cancer. However, even when confronted by these illnesses, we can achieve the maximum level of wellness through nutrition and exercise. (By the way, after supplementing my diet with fish oil concentrate and selenium, the pain in my joint disappeared.)

Well-being is all about getting the most out of life, no matter what your age or state of physical health. Strive for it! Through good eating habits and the power of nutritional therapy, you can increase your level of well-being and extend your years of fulfilled living.

You are Unique

You are special. There is no one else like you. As a consequence, you and your nutritional requirements are unique. You have a unique genetic profile. No one else has had the same social experiences, has the same eating patterns or bouts of illness. Are you married? Do you have any children? Do you work in an office all day? Is your best friend a smoker? The combination of these and other factors in your background and current environment make you absolutely unique, even if you are an identical twin.

Your life and your body are constantly changing, and the foods and supplements you enjoy today may not be the best choice for you next month or a year from now. Knowing what makes you unique, and how to meet your personal nutritional requirements, will help you to achieve maximum well-being. Why is this?

Think for a moment about the massive adjustments that occurred in your body during the rapid growth between infancy and childhood, or during the years of puberty. All that time the processes transforming your body were shifting and rebalancing the amount and combination of nutrients it required from the food you ate. The same is true after you reach adulthood. Pregnancy and breast-feeding are two obvious times when your nutritional requirements change dramatically.

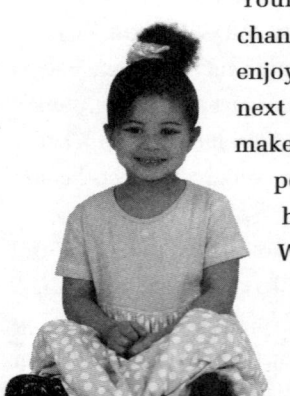

ABOVE CHILDREN NEED SPECIFIC NUTRIENTS TO HELP THEM GROW.

Your unique food requirements alter as your life unfolds. The stress caused by moving house, a death or illness in the family, the challenge of a new job, or a new baby in the household alters your need for nutrients. So too do an injury or infection, a period of sustained physical exertion, a new medication, or a major illness such as diabetes or asthma. All these significantly modify your nutritional requirements. Recognizing any symptoms of dietary imbalance that occur with change, and taking steps to select foods and use supplements that meet your new condition, will help you keep your body in balance.

There will be times when you may not be able to manipulate food choices to your best advantage, as the underlying nutritional consequences of your unique life pattern may be too complex for you to understand. This is when it is wise to seek help from a nutritional therapist (see Chapter 10).

Your Changing Need for Food and Nutrients

The following are general guidelines for good nutrition during special periods in your life. If you have symptoms that worry you, seek help from an expert. Details about foods and nutrients mentioned are found in Chapter 5: What Food Contains.

PREGNANCY

To enhance fertility, enjoy a balanced diet, reduce the amount of caffeine and alcohol you drink and avoid excessive dieting and exercise. Substitute plant for animal protein. Increase folic acid intake by sprinkling wheatgerm or oatgerm on food: this will also increase your intake of the B-complex vitamins and vitamin E. Eat more oily fish, and fruits and vegetables rich in antioxidant vitamins. Eat foods rich in zinc and selenium. Use more seeds and nuts in your cooking. Pumpkin seeds and Brazil nuts are good sources of zinc and selenium. Use seed and nut oils rather than animal fat in your cooking.

During pregnancy, follow the above suggestions and increase the amount of fruits and vegetables eaten. Enjoy sprouted seeds each day, especially alfalfa. Eliminate alcohol from your diet, and drink plenty of bottled or filtered water to flush toxins from your kidneys. Significantly reduce your salt intake. While breast-feeding, follow this regime, and avoid any foods to which you are sensitive. To protect your baby, also remove any well-known allergens, such as peanuts, from your diet.

RIGHT PREGNANT WOMEN NEED TO BE PARTICULARLY CAREFUL ABOUT THEIR NUTRITIONAL INTAKE.

THE MENOPAUSE

Begin with a balanced diet, low in animal fats and salt. Cut back on refined sugars and drink plenty of filtered or bottled water. Eat plenty of lean meat, oily fish and shellfish. Use nut and seed oils. Except for a tiny amount of butter used to flavour food, eliminate animal fat from your diet. Enjoy soya-based foods such as tofu, soya milk and miso. Substitute yams for potatoes in your evening meal at least twice a week. Add golden linseed to your baking: examine the various products on the market and see which fits best into your style of cooking. (Soya, yams and linseed contain oestrogen-like substances that many think help control the symptoms of menopause.) Eat plenty of fresh fruit and vegetables to provide vitamins and minerals, and the fibre needed for a healthy bowel.

There are herbal remedies and food supplements available to aid you through the menopause. If you are concerned about what you need, consult an expert.

AGEING

Starting at about 40 years of age, women should follow the menopause diet. Also consider taking additional vitamins A, C and E, and Evening Primrose Oil (EPO). In addition, many people find a good quality multivitamin each day increases their feeling of well-being and resistance to infection.

Your body's nutritional requirements change as its digestive and metabolic processes slow down. The capacity to perform certain vital chemical processes becomes sluggish, and the tissues fail to receive substances they need to function normally. An important example of this is the transformation of linoleic acid, an essential fat, into gamma-linoleic acid (GLA), needed for building cellular structures and for intercellular communication. A good way to avoid the harmful consequences of this natural part of the ageing process is to provide the body with a rich source of GLA, such as EPO or Borage oil. Also eat oily fish, which provide other essential fatty acids needed for a healthy heart, strong bones and flexible joints.

Men do not need to fine-tune their diet to the same extent as women during their middle years because they do not experience the same drastic hormonal changes. However, to stay healthy men should avoid obesity and enjoy a balanced diet built around low-fat protein, a mixture of grains and legumes, and plenty of fresh fruits and vegetables. Men will also benefit from eating fish oil and consuming GLA as they grow older.

Sperm production can be improved by including oysters and other zinc-rich foods in your diet, such as offal, shellfish and pumpkin seeds. Vitamin E in combination with zinc has been shown to aid normal prostate function, and therefore reduce night-time urinary frequency. These supplements are also thought to enhance sex drive, although eliminating the lifestyle problems of excessive alcohol consumption, lack of exercise and obesity can often do far more for sexual interest and function than dietary manipulation.

In addiction, an ever-increasing number of research reports indicate that substances in soya beans and soya products reduce the risk of developing prostate cancer.

DURING ILLNESS

Your nutritional requirements greatly alter during illness for the following reasons:

- Metabolic processes slow down during illness. Food supplements are useful in filling the gaps between what you eat and what your body requires for healing.
- Various pharmaceutical drugs compete with normal body functions for nutrients, thus creating a greater demand.
- Food intake changes, sometimes reducing the amounts of certain nutrient-rich foods from the diet.
- The amount of water required increases with fever, and to remove toxins from the body.
- Antibiotics and other drugs can affect the balance of healthy bacteria in the digestive system; live yoghurt, certain commercial preparations, and help from a nutritional therapist may help.

- Tissues break down, increasing the need for protein.
- The immune system is activated, and needs more foods containing zinc and antioxidant vitamins and minerals. (See pp.87–88 for more information on the immune system.)

ABOVE EATING LIVE YOGHURT CAN HELP RETURN THE DIGESTIVE SYSTEM TO BALANCE DURING OR AFTER ILLNESS.

GENERAL TIPS FOR HEALTHY EATING

Drink at least two or three pints of water a day. Bottled or filtered is best. Your body needs water to maintain normal fluid balance, flush out toxins and maintain a healthy digestive system.

Enjoy a diet based on vegetables, fruit and complex carbohydrates, balanced with nuts, seeds, and protein foods. Remember to chew nuts and seeds well. For protein, enjoy fish and poultry. For most people, the right balance of calories from major nutrients is: carbohydrates 45%; protein 30%; fats 25%. Saturated fats, however, should be kept to a minimum.

Choose organic products. You body needs purity. Modern agricultural methods and food-processing introduce man-made chemicals that play no part in the delicately balanced natural processes of life. Avoid them. Look for labels that state that food was grown according to the strict rules of organic farming.

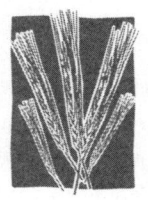

HOW NUTRITIONAL THERAPY WORKS

CHAPTER THREE

Your body is made of many parts. Atoms join to molecules, molecules join and become cells, and cells combine to form tissues and organs. Each part performs a specific function. The most basic of these parts come from the air you breathe and the food and water you consume. In your body's most perfect condition, all parts are in balance. Increasing age, illness and injury cause imbalances that can be corrected or improved by nutritional therapy.

How Poor Nutrition Causes Illness

An unbalanced diet may lead to ill health. To understand the reason for this, imagine an enormous building, a factory, producing jigsaw puzzles of pictures called Perfect Health. The factory is divided into billions of little rooms, each containing a team of experts who are cutting and hammering and pasting at a frantic pace to produce multiple copies of just one part of that massive puzzle. (Obviously, the factory is your body, and its rooms are the billions of cells working together to make it function. We sometimes forget that hundreds of thousands of complex life-sustaining biochemical processes take place in each of the body's cells every day.)

In some ways, all the expert teams in the factory are the same: they all require some of the same raw materials. Let's imagine that these are glue and wood (say – protein and food energy), and they all need to have these materials delivered to them in a timely and orderly fashion. After puzzle pieces are complete, they need to be transported away for assembly, and waste from the production process must be removed on a regular basis. (In the same manner, cell products and waste also must be carried away.)

But these teams of experts also have unique requirements. Let us imagine that gold paint is needed for special puzzle pieces. Distinctive hammers are required to produce individually curved edges found on only three or four pieces. When all the pieces are accurately made, and there are no delays in their manufacture, the result is a beautiful whole: that picture of Perfect Health. (In this fanciful example, the gold paint and distinctive hammers are essential minerals and vitamins required by groups of cells.)

Now, imagine what happens when the management of supplies fails. The deliveries to the factory dwindle, not providing enough glue and gold paint, and there are no new hammers. Work is disrupted. Clever teams may use or build substitutes to complete their puzzle pieces, but only for a time. Soon the pieces become misshapen, function poorly – and finally – are not produced at all.

Imagine that the factory's disposal system becomes blocked. Waste builds up, clogging the distribution routes for delivery of raw materials and the pick-up of finished puzzle pieces. First on one floor, and then throughout the factory, individual teams stop work. The factory may still be able to produce puzzles, but the picture is jagged, unclear, and may be missing entire sections.

That is the way nutrition works: food is the source of raw materials that 'feeds' the factory that is your body. If nutrients are missing, or the balance of nutrients is abnormal, things go astray and illness results. Sometimes the consequences are severe, causing life-threatening nutritional deficiencies, such as scurvy. In our over-fed but under-nourished Western societies, the results of unbalanced nutrition are often slow and insidious. As in the imaginary factory, the diet fails to provide as much of a specific nutrient as the body requires, but the body is resilient: it copes and finds a way around the deficiency. Over time, however, tissue changes occur and these lead to debilitating chronic illnesses. Consuming an unhealthy balance of fats, for example, can cause changes in arterial walls and cells structures, which, over time, may lead to cardiovascular disease and cancer. The human body needs specific nutrients that act as building blocks in a healthy body. When amounts are too low, or not in balance with one another, good health suffers.

ABOVE WESTERN DIETS OFTEN FEATURE HIGH-FAT, PROCESSED FOODS THAT HAVE LITTLE NUTRITIONAL VALUE.

There is a second important aspect of nutritional therapy: using the healing quality of natural compounds in plants. These compounds are often referred to in magazine and newspaper articles as 'phytochemicals'. They can improve well-being by helping your body to fight disease.

Let us go back to our metaphorical factory. Say that everything is running smoothly; then disaster strikes. There is a fire, or a bus crashes into the side of the building. It is true that by adjusting the flow of supplies and upgrading the disposal system, problems caused by these events may be corrected within the factory. But more is needed. Sometimes a totally new material can be brought into the factory that can speed up the reconstruction of the building, or clean up noxious waste after the fire.

Applying these ideas to the human body, the liver builds up toxins over time; many nutritional therapists use special diets to help remove the unhealthy waste. A variety of environmental factors increase body levels of damaging molecules called free radicals, and powerful plant antioxidants – such as lycopene in tomatoes – help deactivate them. Substances in cranberries, blueberries, red grapes and blackberries have strong antibacterial and antiviral properties, and can help control potentially dangerous infections by attacking invading organisms. Using cranberry juice to help control bladder infections (cystitis) is a well-known example. There are powerful cancer fighters in foods such as cauliflower, green tea, broccoli, soya beans and certain mushrooms.

None of these natural plant chemicals plays any role in what we think of as the 'normal' biological processes that keep the human body up and running. But they are powerful tools in the practice of nutritional therapy, and are causing great excitement among other healing professions as well.

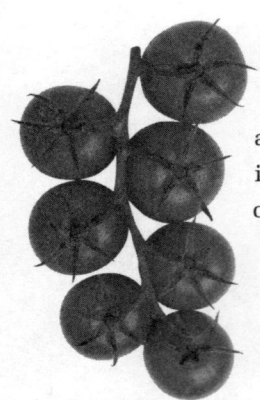

ABOVE TOMATOES CONTAIN ANTIOXIDANTS THAT COUNTERACT THE DAMAGING EFFECT OF FREE RADICALS.

That is the essence of nutritional therapy: balancing essential nutrients and choosing foods to enjoy in ways that take advantage of the healing compounds they contain. We all want to be healthy. By knowing the fundamental facts of nutrition you can work towards that goal and help your body recover from many common complaints. Following the rules of good nutrition gives you remarkable control over your own health.

THE TOOLS OF NUTRITIONAL THERAPY

Nutritional therapists use a variety of treatment methods to help clients. Frequently these involve a modified diet and the inclusion of food supplements to replace specific nutrients depleted by illness or poor diet. But other methods are just as important. These include diets that remove toxins from the body, eliminate allergens from the diet, and re-balance the intake of food to enhance digestion and

CASE STUDY

Sarah was a committed vegan, avoiding all chicken, red meat, fish, poultry, eggs and dairy products. Instead, she enjoyed a diet high in fresh fruit, red and green leafy vegetables, and roasted root vegetables. Soya products were avoided because Sarah worried about the genetic modification of soya, and had not liked the soya protein milk formula that her mother prepared when she was a child.

Proud of her slim body, Sarah ate very modest servings of either rice or beans each day. She looked well, felt well, and was sure she was getting enough of all the nutrients she needed, especially vitamins and slow-release complex carbohydrates. Then, after about a year, she seemed to lose energy, and began noticing that her hair and skin were looking dull. Still more worrying, she seemed to be suffering an unending series of minor infections.

She sought help, and was told she was probably not eating the right balance of food to provide all the essential amino acids her body needed to maintain a healthy immune system and build strong body tissues. One problem was that she ate rice and beans at separate times. Each contains essential protein she needs, but neither contains all the essential protein she needs. She was told to mix beans and grain at the same meal: essential amino acids need to be absorbed at the same time to be effective. A deficiency in one amino acid is the same as having a deficiency in all amino acids: they work in balance and harmony. Sarah was also encouraged to include soya products in her diet. New soya products containing non-genetically modified beans are now available.

The nutritional therapist that Sarah consulted pointed out that Sarah's old diet was probably not providing all the vitamin B12 she needed for healthy red blood cells and nerves. She was advised to add fortified cereals and yeast extract to her diet. Six months after her modified diet, Sarah was once again a slim picture of health.

reduce gastric stagnation. Depending on a person's unique combination of symptoms, a therapist may combine treatment methods. These methods may change during the course of treatment. As is true in all methods of healing, finding the right therapy is sometimes a matter of trial and error: a patient is diagnosed, treatment is prescribed, the healing process is observed, and the treatment methods modified to increase and enhance healing.

The following section briefly describes methods used in nutritional therapy. Some of these methods are best used in the hands of a trained expert.

MODIFYING EATING HABITS

Your health and well-being can be improved by learning new eating patterns. Diet modification can increase levels of vital nutrients, eliminate allergens and stomach irritants, and increase your energy levels. How is this done? Simply by shifting the balance of foods eaten. Even small modifications in the choice of foods can make a remarkable difference. For example, a diet low in foods containing complex carbohydrates and high in refined sugars can cause unpleasant symptoms, such as feelings of dizziness and weakness. In healthy people, simply by eating more pasta, potatoes and pulses, and reducing the amount of sugary foods and beverages, these symptoms can be avoided.

WEIGHT-LOSS DIETS

Excessive weight gain is a major problem for many people in Western cultures. Obesity is linked

LEFT SIMPLE CHANGES TO YOUR DIET, SUCH AS CONSUMING MORE PROTEIN-RICH PULSES, CAN HELP TO INCREASE YOUR ENERGY LEVELS AND GENERAL WELL-BEING.

with an increased risk of developing major illness, such as cancer, heart disease, high blood pressure and stroke. We should shed unwanted and dangerous flab by burning more food energy – calories – than we eat. Exercising regularly plays an important role in maintaining a healthy weight, as does watching what you eat.

Sensible diets do three things:
- Reduce the total calories consumed during a day to less than an average person's body would burn during the same time.
- Provide a healthy blend of nutrients. For example, a good diet will contain little saturated animal fat, but provide adequate fat from fish, nuts and seeds.
- Provide enough fibre and bulk so that you will not feel hungry.

A long list of diets have been devised over the years. Some of them are dangerously silly: the egg and grapefruit diet, for example, is one that has little nutritional merit, as are diets high in protein and very low in sources of carbohydrate. Remember that factory discussed earlier? If a diet does not provide a balanced flow of nutrients, think twice before you try it.

HIGH-PROTEIN RAPID WEIGHT LOSS DIETS

High-protein diets deserve mention because of their new popularity. They place emphasis on foods containing very limited amounts of carbohydrate (such as beef, fish and chicken) and the exclusion of starchy foods, including those based on grains. Proponents of these diets claim that they have special fat-reducing powers, although this is not substantiated by scientific evidence. Many people probably lose weight because the permitted foods are rich and filling, reducing the total numbers of calories consumed. High-protein diets are not recommended because they contain limited fibre needed for a healthy bowel, place stress on the liver and kidneys, encourage calcium loss from the body, and many are high in potentially harmful saturated fats.

CORRECTING DEFICIENCIES

Deficiencies can occur when the body does not receive all the nutrients that it needs. These deficiencies can be corrected by modifying the selection of foods eaten, or by taking food

CASE STUDY

Patsy ate three meals a day and, conscious of her weight, did not eat snacks between meals or after dinner. Her diet was well balanced, and she had no physical complaints, although she was concerned about the extra half-stone in weight that she had gained after the birth of her second child. Patsy tried cutting down on the amount of food that she ate, but found that by the time she reached the supper table in the evening, she was extremely hungry. Caring for two children under five, and helping her husband run their small farm, also consumed a lot of Patsy's energy. She met a nutritional therapist through a friend, and asked for advice. A simple change in eating habits proved to work rapidly and well. Instead of concentrating her total intake of calories during three meals, spaced over a period of about twelve hours, Patsy was told to snack – to graze – throughout the day on foods high in complex carbohydrates. By choosing apples and other fruits instead of cakes, and oat and fruit bars rather than ice cream to satisfy her sweet tooth, and by enjoying more low-fat meats, such as fish and chicken breast, she actually reduced her total calorie intake, despite seeming to eat all day long.

Patsy's unwanted weight disappeared in a matter of weeks without the misery of a restrictive diet. Better still, she seemed to regain the stamina she had before the baby was born. Grazing gave her a constant flow of energy that kept the hunger pangs at bay, and gave her the lift she needed to enjoy life again.

supplements. An example of an important nutritional deficiency that can be corrected by either means involves the mineral selenium. This mineral is part of the natural antioxidant system in the body, and has been linked with reduced rates of certain cancers and heart disease. In some parts of the world, levels of selenium are so low that experts believe the population to be at risk. Children in China are known to develop heart failure because of a deficiency in this essential mineral, for example. Supplements can be used to correct selenium deficiency, or food choices can be improved, including more liver, whole grains (grown in selenium-rich soil), Brazil nuts and shellfish.

DETOXIFICATION

Over time, harmful chemicals in food, water and the air we breathe collect and concentrate in the liver and in fat tissues. In addition, the body produces its own toxic substances, especially when we are under stress. A few symptoms of toxic build-up include a sluggish feeling, an inability to concentrate, low energy levels, chronic constipation, and itchy skin with no apparent cause.

The body tries to expel the toxins responsible, but sometimes fails. An answer is to take a detoxification programme. These can be very brief or last as long as a fortnight. Some focus only on dietary changes, and others involve cleansing the colon.

If you are interested in trying a detoxification programme, read several sources on this subject and seek advice. However, a simple programme to get you started is to eat only fruit and drink only water or herbal tea from the time you get up until lunchtime; then return to your usual diet. Many people find that this does wonders.

ABOVE DRINKING PLENTY OF WATER TO HELP FLUSH OUT ACCUMULATED TOXINS IS AN IMPORTANT PART OF DETOXIFICATION REGIMES.

FOOD COMBINING (THE HAY DIET)

In the early 1900s, Dr William Hay, an American, developed an eating plan that he claimed would help natural healing. He linked arthritis, constipation, indigestion and skin conditions with unhealthy chemical balance in the body, and he stressed eating foods that make the blood alkaline (such as fruits, vegetables and milk). Foods that raised the acid level (such as citrus fruits, meat and carbohydrates) were to be eaten in smaller quantities. In addition he stated that protein-rich foods and carbohydrate-rich foods should not be eaten at the same meal; that carbohydrate and protein meals should be separated by at least four hours; that fruits and vegetables – including leafy greens – should form the majority of foods eaten; that animal protein and carbohydrate should be eaten in small amounts; and that refined sugar and processed foods should be avoided.

There is no scientific rationale behind this diet. However, many people with chronic stomach complaints find that they feel better when following the Hay diet. Followers of the Hay diet often also experience weight loss, but this may be because they tend to eat little fat and one or two carbohydrate-free meals during the day.

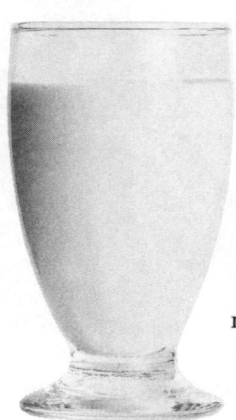

Modern adaptations of the Hay diet are known as food-combining diets. These are healthy because they are high in nutrient-rich foods and contain little fat and protein.

HYPOALLERGENIC DIETS

A hypoallergenic diet is a prescribed eating regimen that is completely devoid of one or more foods that have been shown to cause an allergic reaction.

Sensitivities to various foods are recognised as a cause of illness. Sometimes these sensitivities produce such

ABOVE MILK IS OFTEN CONSIDERED TO BE HEALTHY, BUT MANY PEOPLE ARE ALLERGIC OR INTOLERANT TO IT.

Case Study

Martin is a gardener, and because he likes growing and eating tomatoes, red peppers, aubergine and potatoes – all members of the nightshade plant family – the late summer is a time to enjoy salads made of sliced peppers and tomatoes, warmed by the sun, and picked fresh from his garden. For dinner, his wife prepares dishes rich with these flavourful vegetables. However, as Martin grows older, he is noticing that his hands itch and redden when he peels potatoes, or cleaned peppers for roasting. And, his lips seem to tingle after enjoying a ripe red tomato. After eating a hearty meal of these favourite foods, he feels somewhat light-headed and fuzzy. On advice from an expert nutritionist, he decided to avoid eating his favourite vegetables, and to give his bountiful crop away to his neighbours.

The members of the nightshade family mentioned above are not true vegetables, but fruits. They originated in South America, although they are usually associated with the cuisine of the Mediterranean region. They all contain a toxin called solanine – although its concentration is lowest in red-skinned potatoes. In high levels, this toxin can cause headaches, mental confusion, diarrhoea and vomiting. Solanine and other strong compounds in the nightshade family can be somewhat neutralised by roasting, frying, and cooking with salt or miso.

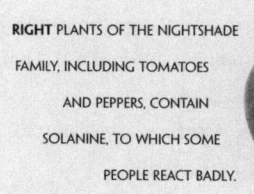

RIGHT PLANTS OF THE NIGHTSHADE FAMILY, INCLUDING TOMATOES AND PEPPERS, CONTAIN SOLANINE, TO WHICH SOME PEOPLE REACT BADLY.

severe allergic reactions that an individual goes into shock. Other food sensitivities, or allergies, are less obvious, particularly in adults. Foods that can cause sensitivity include: peanuts, gluten (a protein in wheat and some other grains), dairy products (particularly from cow's milk), vegetables of the nightshade family (including peppers, potatoes, tomatoes and aubergines), various types of seafood, yeast, eggs and citrus fruits.

Allergy to cows' milk is common, although frequently unsuspected. Human infants can develop an allergy to milk protein that is so severe the child may exhibit projectile vomiting. (This is one of the reasons that 'breast is best'.) In adults, milk sensitivity can take many forms, including bloating, loose stools, gas, belching, stomach pain, and, most surprisingly to many people, a release of

Case Study

Jerome was a retired ambulance driver who suffered from migraine headaches and gastric pain. To ease the pain, his doctor prescribed first aspirin, and then a compound containing ibuprofin. While both help the pain, they also caused gastric irritation and, eventually, bleeding. As part of his treatment, Jerome was referred to the hospital nutrition clinic, where he was placed on a bland diet. To his surprise, after a few weeks his headaches disappeared. When he was allowed to eat a wider selection of food, however, he noticed that the headaches returned. Jerome reported this to the nutritionist at the clinic. She showed him how to maintain a food diary, and make notes on what he ate and when he suffered from migraines. He discovered his headaches appeared up to 72 hours after eating blue-veined cheeses (such as Roquefort), chocolate and citrus fruits. Once this was known, Jerome adjusted his eating habits by eliminating these foods. After about six months, he suffered neither migraines nor gastric pain.

excessive mucus in the respiratory tract. By identifying this allergy, and removing all foods containing cow's milk from the diet, relief can be rapid. Good substitutes are fortified soya milk, and products made with goats' or ewes' milk.

The diagnosis of a food allergy through an elimination diet should be undertaken with professional supervision. Methods vary, but in general all the foods possibly responsive for symptoms are removed from the diet for a fortnight and signs of improvement are monitored. After this cleansing period, and beginning with tap water, foods are introduced one at a time at two-day intervals. If there is a reaction to a new food, it is eliminated. This procedure is continued until all the causes of symptoms have been identified. This process takes time, and professional guidance is needed to insure that a healthy diet is maintained despite strict food limitations.

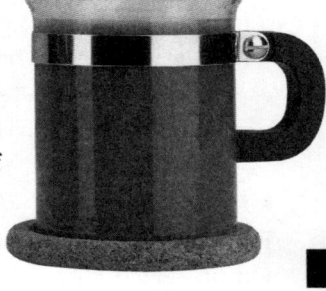

ABOVE REMOVING CAFFEINE FROM YOUR DIET CAN BE A SIMPLE WAY OF IMPROVING YOUR HEALTH.

A simple exclusion diet to try is eliminating food and drink containing caffeine from your food choices. Caffeine is a powerful substance that many nutritionists believe can have negative health effects. Consuming too much can make you feel jumpy, cause insomnia and migraine headaches. It may also accelerate the loss of minerals from bone. Removing caffeine from your diet may help to improve your state of well-being by reducing stress and eliminating the symptoms of trembling hands, racing heart and the feeling that your head will explode because of nerves. As caffeine is mildly habit-forming, some people find that they have headaches and generally feel terrible when they suddenly stop drinking and eating all foods containing this natural stimulant. If you think reducing your caffeine intake may help you, remember to cut out all cola drinks as well as coffee.

JUICING

Juicing is an effective means of concentrating nutrients. By pulping and then squeezing fresh fruit and vegetables, the bulky fibre and pith that make up much of the structure of foods from plants is removed and natural juices flow free. Different combinations of foods result in different blends of nutrients, so there are a number of juicing 'recipes' available. For people who require concentrated natural nutrients, balanced as they are in nature, juicing provides a quick and effective means of improving your diet. You should not forget, however, that the fibrous parts of fruits and vegetables play an important part in the normal cleansing of your bowel, and pith – especially in citrus fruit – contains phytochemicals that help protect you against serious illness.

MONO-DIETS AND FASTING

Fasting is part of an ancient tradition of self-cleansing and mental purification. Today, for curing illness, fasting is more likely to be recommended by a naturopath than a nutritional therapist. It is reasoned that if a person refrains from food, and drinks only water, the body can expend all its resources on healing itself, rather than on the energy-consuming processes of digestion and metabolism of food.

There are many different ways to fast. Some involve drinking juices during abstinence from solid food. Others allow one selected food to be eaten: grapes are a typical choice.

Fasting should be done under supervision, as it can have serious side-effects. In addition, fasting is not a sensible way to lose weight; any weight lost during a fast is usually replaced very quickly after resuming a normal diet.

ANTI-CANDIDA DIETS

The overgrowth of a yeast normally found in the human body, called Candida albicans, causes a common illness known as candidiasis, thrush or moniliasis. Overgrowth, or infection, usually affects the vagina, the mouth and areas of moist skin. Many sufferers of candidiasis experience a cluster of symptoms, which can include headaches, bloating, wind, persistent fatigue, itching and mild depression.

Candida overgrowth can also cause gastric illness in people suffering from an impaired immune system. Candida's growth is usually kept under control by normal bacteria in the body, but when antibiotic drugs destroy this protection, the fungus' reproduction is unrestricted. Mental and physical stress, long illnesses, asthma, recurrent infections, dietary deficiencies in important micronutrients, and damage to the immune system set the stage for the abnormal spread of the candida fungus. Other circumstances promoting the growth of Candida are oral contraceptives, the normal hormonal changes in the female body, and diabetes.

Candidiasis can be treated by keeping damp skin dry (avoiding nappy-rash, for example), avoiding cross-infection through sexual contact, and the use of anti-fungal creams and pills. Approaching the problem through nutritional changes is an important mode of care alone or in combination with any of the previously mentioned methods.

Enjoying foods that support the immune system can help control this condition. The anti-Candida diet permits no ingestion of any sweetened food or drink high in natural sugars: this includes fruits such as dried apricots and bananas. Sufferers are encouraged to eat plenty of soya, garlic, onions and leeks, and extra-virgin olive oil. As food allergies are frequently associated with candidiasis, a hypoallergenic diet is often prescribed along with these changes in food choices.

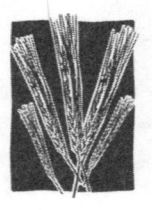

DIGESTION: TURNING FOOD INTO MOLECULES

CHAPTER FOUR

The digestive system is the vital core of your well-being upon which all the body's processes depend. No bone can grow, no tissue can repair itself; and no thought or dream can occur without the presence of vital nutrients that drive the processes. These nutrients come packaged as food, which must be broken down and extracted before they are made available to the body's cells. This is the task of the digestive system. The digestive organs are highly complex systems that carry out many physical and chemical activities. If, for any reason, these activities are thwarted, or occur too quickly or too slowly, major alterations in the flow of nutrients to your body occur that can set the stage for health problems. You can eat the most perfectly balanced diet in the world, but unless your digestive system works normally, you run the risk of nutrient imbalance. For this reason, nutrition therapy places considerable emphasis on achieving and maintaining a healthy digestive system.

Why should we be concerned with the process of digestion? Because if anything affects or disrupts digestion, it limits the amount of nutrients available to the body. Anything from inadequate time spent chewing, to antibiotics that destroy the normal balance of bacterial flora in the lower gut, will disrupt the digestive process. If you suffer from an illness, for example Irritable Bowel Syndrome, your whole body's nutritional status needs attention. If you contract food poisoning, and your digestive system is invaded by an organism that gives you diarrhoea, your body's nutrient and fluid systems will be disrupted. If your body fails to absorb the necessary balance of vitamins, you could run the risk of deficiency disease (see pp.86–87). That is why much of nutritional therapy deals with feeding, protecting and restoring the digestive system.

The digestive system consists of a delicately balanced and highly active group of organs. When placed under stress, it signals a warning. It is not unusual to experience occasional belching, flatulence, mild gastric discomfort, constipation or diarrhoea. Common reasons for digestive distress include eating foods that cause flatulence and gas, eating too much or too little food over a period of time, not drinking enough water, eating contaminated food, not chewing food adequately, stress, smoking, and the action of medications and drugs. Symptoms will often disappear by using simple self-help methods. When such symptoms occur repeatedly, however, it suggests that something more sinister is happening within the digestive tract. Diagnosing digestive problems is not easy because symptoms can have more than one cause. If you try self-help methods and find they fail to eradicate the problem, seek professional guidance. Many people – especially men – tend to ignore the danger signals of chronic digestive problems. By doing so, they risk their good health.

THE DIGESTIVE SYSTEM

The digestive system consists of one muscular tube that begins at the mouth and ends with the rectum. The structure and size of this tube varies to form the oesophagus, the stomach and the intestines.

Muscular contractions (peristalsis) flow down the tube, mixing food and moving it along. The mass (bolus) of food moves onwards from the mouth. Special glands along the way introduce enzymes and other chemicals that break down the complex molecules of food into simple molecules that can be absorbed by the body. These simple molecules are the nutrients on which all life processes depend. Minerals and vitamins are released and absorbed into the bloodstream. Starches become sugar; proteins become amino acids, and fats become smaller derivatives. Much of the food eaten as fruits and vegetables consists of fibrous bulk, which the digestive system cannot break down. This fibrous material gradually forms a mass that aids the removal of waste from the body.

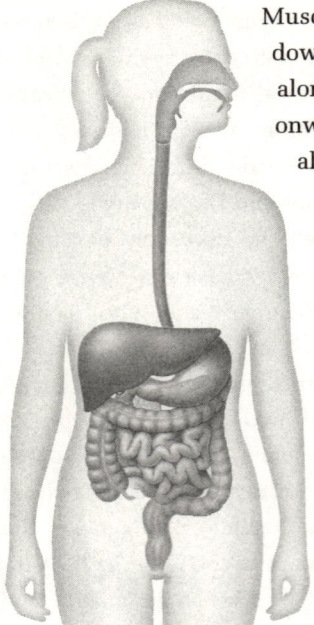

ABOVE THE DIGESTIVE SYSTEM IS BASICALLY A MUSCULAR TUBE STARTING WITH THE MOUTH AND LEADING TO THE RECTUM.

Digestion begins in the mouth with the process of chewing. Food is ground down and broken up into small pieces by the teeth. As food is chewed, saliva is released by glands near the mouth. This contains an enzyme, amylase, which begins the process of reducing starch molecules into sugar: the better food is chewed, the more complete this early stage of digestion. (It is worth remembering that small pieces of food are easier to digest than large, so even when you are in a hurry, you can save your stomach distress by taking time to chew your food well before swallowing.)

Swallowed food passes into the oesophagus, where the rhythmic waves of peristalsis continue to mix the food as it moves down and into a large muscular 'bulge' in the digestive tract: the stomach. The muscles here knead and squeeze the partially digested food and press it against the mucus-coated membrane covering its lining. Millions of tiny, highly specialised glands cover this lining, and secrete various substances: mucus (which protects the stomach from digesting itself); digestive enzymes that begin the process of dismantling proteins; hydrochloric acid; and 'intrinsic factor', which is essential for the absorption of vitamin B12 in the small intestine. The stomach is a grinding and mixing machine; only certain drugs and alcohol are absorbed at this stage. After about five hours, the partially digested food moves on into the small intestine, from where almost all nutrients are absorbed.

The small intestine is a coiled muscular tube almost twenty-five feet (eight metres) long. It has three parts: the duodenum, jejunum and ileum. Fluids from the bile duct (which is attached to the liver) and the pancreas flow into the duodenum (the top part of the small intestine) and neutralize the highly acidic matter entering from the stomach. A change from acid to alkaline is needed before digestive enzymes can function further. Pancreatic juices contain enzymes involved in the digestion of proteins, carbohydrates and fats. Bile facilitates the digestion of fats by acting as a kind of detergent; it also carries waste from the liver into the intestine for disposal later.

Peristalsis carries the partially digested food on into the jejunum and ileum, where it comes into contact with millions of tiny finger-like protrusions called villi. These increase the area of contact between the now quite fluid material being digested and the intestinal wall. Glands at the base of the villi add substances similar to that released by the pancreas.

It is in the small intestine where most of the absorption of amino acids, sugar, short-chain fats, vitamins and minerals takes place. These substances are absorbed through the villi and carried by the bloodstream to the portal vein of the liver. Longer chain fats enter the body through the lymphatic system of the small intestine. From here, what remains travels on to the large intestine, where fluid is absorbed. No digestion occurs here, as there are no villi, but a host of bacteria add to the bulk of the waste. After some hours, the waste from digestion is passed from the body. The absorption process takes about nine hours; waste may spend from six to twenty-fours hours in the large intestine.

> ### THE IMPORTANCE OF THE LIVER
>
> No discussion of digestion is complete without mentioning the largest internal organ of the human body: the liver. The liver produces bile, necessary for the digestion of fats. It converts beta-carotene into vitamin A, which it stores. It stores glycogen – a form of carbohydrate that helps to sustain blood-sugar levels. The liver also constructs factors needed for normal blood-clotting, enzymes and cholesterol. Of particular interest in our polluted world, the liver plays a crucial role in the detoxification of dangerous molecules. For this reason, nutrition therapists use many methods to help 'detoxify' the liver.

METABOLISM

The processes in which nutrients from food are dealt with once inside the body is called metabolism. There are two phases to metabolism: catabolism, which is the process of breaking down large molecules; and anabolism, which involves the building up of new molecules. Both catabolism and anabolism are processes that occur continually. Catabolism frequently results in the release of energy. (The simple sugar glucose is broken down into energy, water and carbon dioxide, a waste product.) Anabolism usually requires energy.

'Metabolic rate' is the speed at which energy from food is burned by the body. Food energy not burned is stored as fat. Several factors affect the metabolic rate, but the most important is a hormone produced by the thyroid gland. For normal activity, this gland requires iodine from the diet. (This is an example of how an abnormal level of one nutrient can greatly influence the entire body.)

PROTEIN METABOLISM

A quick review of protein metabolism is a good way to explore how these two aspects of metabolism work together. The body is constantly building protein molecules – for enzymes, for blood fluids, for muscle, for various structural parts of cells, as hormones. In a normal human, there are thousands of individual types, or 'species' of proteins, each having a specific task to perform. Proteins consist of hundreds, even thousands, of basic protein-building units, called amino acids. These are very precisely arranged in long chains. The exacting anabolic process of making protein molecules is constant, although the rate at which some protein chains are made varies with fluctuating conditions in the body as a whole.

Amino acids come from a variety of sources. Some of them come from the diet. A healthy, middle-aged woman should consume approximately 45 grams (two ounces) of pure protein per day. But that is not enough to supply all the millions of amino acids used during that same period of time. This is one of the ways in which catabolism plays an important role. Protein molecules are made, used, and can be broken down into their amino acid units to again be restructured into new protein. The body can even manufacture one type of amino acid from another. But fresh amino acid supplies must also be brought in from outside sources, for two reasons. As one would expect, some protein is used up during the body's processes. More importantly, there are certain amino acids that the body cannot manufacture, and these must come from food. These are called 'essential amino acids' (see p.51).

RIGHT FISH SUCH AS TROUT ARE A GOOD SOURCE OF THE ESSENTIAL AMINO ACIDS.

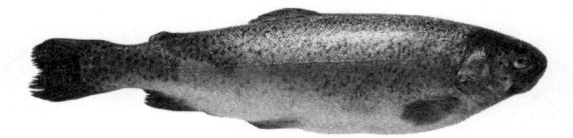

For normal metabolism – including the production of all the specific types of protein molecules that the body needs, adequate supplies of all the essential amino acids must be present. The body will use no substitutes. If even one essential amino acid is in short supply, the body is ultimately protein-deficient.

This story about protein is important because it points out the body's dependence on food – and normal digestion – to provide the full range of nutrients required to maintain good health.

All Things in Moderation

Keep in mind that good and healthy foods can at times cause problems. For example, you may have already experienced the effects of enjoying too much hot curry. But did you know that too much cabbage can cause goitre, and interfere with the activity of the thyroid gland, which is the regulator of our metabolic processes? Or that an excess of nutmeg can be toxic? Rhubarb and spinach contain oxalic acid, which in high doses builds kidney stones. Excessive amounts of liquorice results in high blood pressure; and the solanine in the green part of sprouting potatoes can be toxic. You can have too much of a good thing. The golden rule for a healthy digestive system is moderation.

LEFT CABBAGE CONTAINS MANY VALUABLE NUTRIENTS AND IS BELIEVED TO HAVE ANTICANCER PROPERTIES, BUT AN EXCESS MAY CAUSE GOITRE.

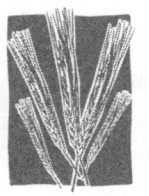

WHAT FOOD CONTAINS

CHAPTER FIVE

Everything you eat and drink contains a blend of only six categories of nutrients required for normal body activity: water, carbohydrates, proteins, fats, minerals and vitamins. This consistency in the basic content of food is remarkable when one considers the vast number of variations in flavours and textures that we find in foods. However, different foods vary widely in the balance of nutrients that they contain. Understanding this is the key to selecting a combination of foods for a healthy diet. To obtain all the nutrients needed for normal growth, energy, muscle movement, brain function and reproduction, a diet should contain a combination of foods from a variety of plants (and animals, if necessary). In addition to these required nutrients, plants also provide substances (phytochemicals) that have been shown to aid the human body in its fight against disease.

Almonds and spinach contain ingredients from the six basic categories, but in very different proportions. Almonds are an excellent source of certain fats that

RIGHT ALMONDS CONTAIN A NUMBER OF VALUABLE FATS, PROTEIN, VITAMINS AND MINERALS.

we need to eat, as well as protein, minerals and vitamins. Spinach contains very small amounts of fats, protein and carbohydrate, but is a rich source of vitamins and minerals. Even the vitamins and minerals in these two foods from plants differ widely. Spinach is a good source of beta-carotene (which the body converts to vitamin A), folic acid and vitamin C. Almonds provide polyunsaturated fats, vitamin E (which works with vitamin C to give protective antioxidant effects), and the B-complex vitamins thiamine, riboflavin and niacin.

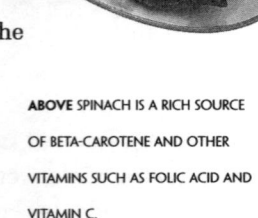

ABOVE SPINACH IS A RICH SOURCE OF BETA-CAROTENE AND OTHER VITAMINS SUCH AS FOLIC ACID AND VITAMIN C.

Oily fish and lean beef share the same types of nutrients, but in different proportions. For example, oily fish is an excellent source of the highly desirable nutrients known as omega-3 fatty acids; beef and other types of red meat contain none of these essential fats. Like beef, fish has a high level of the kind of complete protein needed for human health, but neither mackerel nor lean beef contain carbohydrate. Meat is a good source of iron, like spinach, because this mineral is used in both green plants and red animal muscle as an important component of the natural biological processes that occur in them. By contrast, almonds and mackerel contain very low quantities of iron.

For the body to function normally, you need more of some categories of nutrients than others. The MACRONUTRIENTS (carbohydrates, proteins and fats) make up the bulk of foods you eat, and are the stuff that gives you the energy and building blocks for body growth and repair. But macronutrients alone are not enough. The MICRONUTRIENTS, minerals and vitamins, are needed in much smaller quantities, but are essential for the biological processes in your body that digest and use the food you eat.

MACRONUTRIENTS

WATER
Do not take your need for water for granted. The normal processes of the body require between 2 and 2.5 litres of water per day. Some of this comes from food, especially fruits and vegetables, but most comes from what you drink. Tea, coffee and other caffeinated drinks are no substitute for water, as they have a mild diuretic effect. You should increase your water consumption when working out or perspiring heavily.

CARBOHYDRATE
Carbohydrates, the primary source of food energy, have two forms: simple sugars and complex carbohydrates, which are formed from linked chains of simple sugars. Complex carbohydrates are either starch, like that found in grains and root vegetables, or indigestible fibre. Simple sugars are quickly absorbed into the bloodstream, where they provide energy to the body's cells. Digestible complex carbohydrate must be broken down in the body before its simple sugars can be released and used. Indigestible complex carbohydrates pass through the gut unchanged.

The body works best when a steady flow of sugar to turn into energy is released into the bloodstream. A quick rise in blood sugar levels increases the production of insulin, which drains off the sugar for storage as glycogen in muscle and liver tissue.

Good carbohydrate sources include pasta, rice, cereals, root vegetables and bread.

FIBRE
Fibre is a complex carbohydrate made of long chains of linked simple sugars. However, because of the way these sugars are strung together, the human digestive system is unable to break them down and turn the sugars into energy. Although fibre has no energy, or 'caloric' value, it is nonetheless a vital part of your diet.

Foods high in fibre help to control hunger pangs and appetite because fibre provides bulk in the digestive system. Fibre also helps to control blood sugar levels by slowing the rate at which sugar is released from other complex carbohydrates, and it aids the passage of digested matter from the body. Healthy levels of dietary fibre help to prevent constipation and many bowel problems, including weakening of the bowel wall and cancer of the colon.

There are two kinds of fibre: soluble and insoluble. Insoluble fibre forms bulk that increases the frequency of bowel movements. Soluble fibre, found in oat and soya bran, also provides bulk in the diet, but has the added benefit of lowering blood cholesterol by absorbing and eliminating it from the body.

The Western diet is low in natural fibre. For good health, include at least four fibre-rich foods in your diet every day (approximately 18 grams in total). Good sources are grains, beans and other pulses, root vegetables and fruit. Good sources of soluble fibre include bran (soya and wheat are particularly good), apples and oats. Good sources of insoluble fibre include wholemeal flour, bran, popcorn, barley, rye flour, peas and beans.

A word of caution: do not heap wheat bran on your food as a means of increasing your daily fibre intake. Wheat bran attracts and holds onto vital minerals as they pass through the gut, thus making them unavailable to your body. Too much can irritate the bowel, as it is harsh. It is better to eat beans, lentils, fruit and root vegetables.

PROTEIN

After water, protein is the most abundant substance in the human body. It is necessary for the structure of hair, nails, bones and teeth, the matrix ('living net') that keeps cells and organs in their proper place, for the structure and elasticity of muscle, as part of all body fluids, and for the structure of small, powerful regulatory molecules called enzymes.

The basic building-blocks in protein are the amino acids. Maximum well-being depends on eating an adequate balance of these

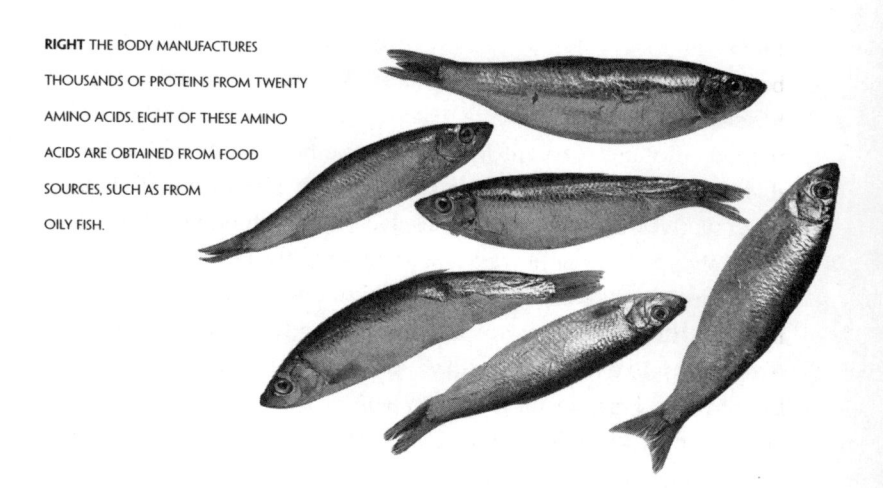

RIGHT THE BODY MANUFACTURES THOUSANDS OF PROTEINS FROM TWENTY AMINO ACIDS. EIGHT OF THESE AMINO ACIDS ARE OBTAINED FROM FOOD SOURCES, SUCH AS FROM OILY FISH.

protein units. Twenty amino acids combine to build healthy tissues; all but eight of these can be manufactured by your body. (There is a ninth that the body sometimes cannot make in adequate quantities to maintain normal tissues.) These eight or sometimes nine amino acids are, therefore, called 'essential amino acids'. Meat contains all of the amino acids that we need. Protein from plant sources vary, and to obtain an adequate balance of all needed amino acids, grains and pulses should be combined.

When you eat protein foods, the amino acids are released through digestion, and are reassembled into proteins that your body needs in order to function. It may surprise you to learn that your body manufactures more than 100,000 different proteins, with functions as diverse as forming antibodies to fight infection, to forming the tough layer that surrounds your brain.

Nutritional therapy takes advantage of the fact that individual amino acids have certain therapeutic functions. Used correctly, lysine can help to prevent and treat the herpes simplex virus. Tryptophan, a precursor of the brain substance serotonin, is used to aid sleep and control mood patterns.

Good protein sources include lean meat, eggs, seafood, soya beans, and beans and cereals.

FATS

Per unit of weight, fat contains more than twice as much energy as either protein or carbohydrate. Fat is part of a more general category of food substances, called lipids. Its basic building blocks are fatty acids. When three fatty acids are attached to a molecule of another lipid – glycerol – they form triglycerides, which are the most common type of fat in the body. In addition to the fat we eat, we make our own. Energy consumed as carbohydrates and protein, and not used by the body, is converted into fat and stored. That is why reducing fat while continuing to eat excessive amounts of carbohydrates may result in weight gain.

Fatty acids are linear molecules that vary in length. They also vary in the degree to which they can potentially contain more hydrogen atoms: if there is no room, they are 'saturated'; if places exist on the molecule where one or more hydrogen atoms can find a place, the fatty acids are classified as monounsaturated, or polyunsaturated, respectively. The most important thing to remember about this is that missing hydrogen atoms make fatty acids biologically active. There are two specific forms of biologically active fatty acid that are essential for human health, and cannot be manufactured by the body: these are the omega-3 and omega-6 fatty acids, and they must come from outside the human body either in food or as food supplements.

From all the diet propaganda, you may think of all fats as bad. However, in addition to being a highly effective way to store the body's energy resources, fats play important roles in structure and physiology. A fatty layer under the skin helps to preserve body heat; fats protect certain internal organs; they form part of every cell membrane; they are a major constituent in the nervous system; and they form part of many of the key hormones and hormone-like substances in the body. We need to eat fat in our diet, but we need to eat the right kinds. Beef burgers and brandy butter will do nothing to meet your need for omega-3 and omega-6 fatty acids; for that, turn to fish and seed oils.

Fats make food more appealing to eat: they have a nice 'mouth-feel', and are added to many processed foods to increase their desirability. For this reason, processed foods present the biggest danger when you try to reduce your fat intake. A balanced diet contains no less than 20% and no more than 33% fat. Remember, saturated fats should constitute no more than 10% of your total fat intake.

Cholesterol is another lipid essential for body structure and biological activity, although the liver produces adequate quantities for normal health. Cholesterol has been given a bad press over the years, but recent research has linked low dietary and blood cholesterol levels with depression.

Good sources of monounsaturated fats are olive oil, avocados and corn oil. Useful sources of polyunsaturated fats are nut oils, corn oil, rapeseed (canola) oil and oily fish such as mackerel and salmon.

For a healthy diet low in saturated fats, you should strictly limit your intake of beef, lamb, pork, butter, hardened margarine, cheese and whole milk.

MICRONUTRIENTS

VITAMINS

Vitamin A (retinol) is found only in animals, which manufacture it from plant substances known as carotenes. The most commonly known of these is beta-carotene. Beta-carotene and other carotenoids are found in brightly coloured edible plants, including carrots, spinach, sweet potatoes, watercress and mangoes. As these substances are converted into vitamin A, deficiency symptoms are the same. Carotenoids are

RIGHT MANGOES AND OTHER ORANGE FRUITS AND VEGETABLES ARE A GOOD SOURCE OF BETA-CAROTENE.

thought to be powerful free-radical quenchers, and thereby act as one source of protection against cancer and heart disease. Vitamin A benefits the skin and mucous membranes of the body, where it helps fight infection. It is also essential for night vision, normal foetal growth, and normal bone formation.

Good sources of vitamin A include: liver, raw carrots, milk, Cheddar cheese and butter.

Note: Vitamin A is one of the few vitamins that can be toxic when taken in very high doses.

The B-vitamins: (Thiamin [B$_1$], Riboflavin [B$_2$], Niacin [B$_3$], Pantothenic acid [B$_5$], Pyridoxine [B$_6$], Cobalamin [B$_{12}$], Folic acid and Biotin.) These water-soluble vitamins play important roles in the release of energy from carbohydrates and fats, and in the metabolism of the brain and nervous system.

Thiamin deficiency can lead to the life-threatening symptoms of beri-beri, and pellagra results from a niacin deficiency.

Normal development of the foetal nervous system requires folic acid, which also plays a vital part in reducing the risk of heart disease.

Improvement in the symptoms of pre-menstrual symptoms, hair loss and dermatitis, osteoarthritis, depression and memory loss has been observed with the use of B-vitamin supplements.

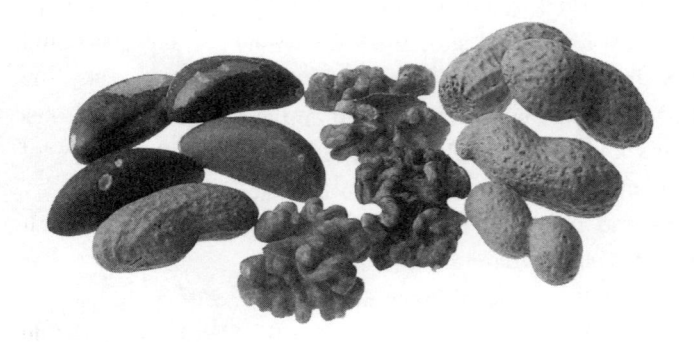

ABOVE NUTS OF ALL VARIETIES ARE EXCELLENT SOURCES OF B VITAMINS. PEANUTS ARE RICH IN NIACIN AND THIAMIN, WHILE BRAZIL NUTS AND WALNUTS ARE A GOOD SOURCE OF FOLATE.

B-vitamins are best consumed from raw foods, as they are lost from food into cooking water and dripping from frozen food.

Good sources include: bread and cereal products, nuts, pulses, green leafy vegetables, milk and meat.

B-complex factors (Choline and Inositol) are not true vitamins because they can be made by the human body. Health benefits can be derived from their use as supplements because they support the activity of the B-vitamins, act as structural parts of cell walls, help prevent abnormal fat build-up in the liver, and may benefit people suffering from atherosclerosis. Choline is part of the nerve transmission substance acetylcholine.

Good food sources are liver, nuts, and pulses.

Vitamin C (ascorbic acid) is a vital part of life processes in all plants and animals. Many living organisms can make this substance within their cells, but humans and certain other animals cannot. The importance of vitamin C is so dynamic that even after decades of study we do not fully understand all of its roles in the human body.

Vitamin C, a water-soluble vitamin, works with vitamin E, a fat-soluble vitamin, in mopping up damaging free radicals (see pp.62–64) in all parts of living tissue. In this role, Vitamin C helps prevent degenerative diseases, including cancer, heart disease and arthritis. It also promotes the production of collagen and the formation of antibodies, facilitates the absorption of iron, encourages normal tissue growth and wound-healing. Severe deficiency of vitamin C results in the disease scurvy.

Vitamin C supplements can help to heal gastric ulcers. However, it is slightly acid, and anyone with a sensitive stomach or who has suffered from ulcers in the past should use a 'buffered' form.

The ingestion of aspirin, birth control pills and cortisone compounds may increase the need for vitamin C. Kidney stone sufferers should not take more than 1 gram per day.

In nature, bioflavonoids (hesperidin, quercetin and rutin) occur with vitamin C, and have been shown to increase the uptake of this vitamin by the body. They have also been shown to have an antihistamine effect, and strengthen blood capillaries.

Good food sources are: blackcurrants, green peppers, mango, cauliflower, cabbage, sweet potato, tomatoes and potatoes. (Oranges and grapefruit contain less vitamin C per 100 grams than either cabbage or cauliflower.) Heat, alkali substances, and exposure to air destroy this nutrient.

Vitamin D: The body converts vitamin D into a hormone that controls calcium balance. Important medical conditions associated with its deficiency are rickets and osteomalacia, and probably osteoporosis. However, deficiency is rare, because in the presence of sunlight, the human body converts cholesterol into vitamin D. People at risk are those who spend little time in sunlight (such as the housebound), or cover their skin completely when going out (such as Muslim women in traditional clothing), or lactating women who are vegans.

Good food sources are: oily fish and dairy products.

Vitamin E: A fat-soluble substance, vitamin E is arguably the most powerful antioxidant nutrient that we receive from food. Once thought to have little benefit for humans, we now know that it reduces the risk of circulatory conditions, including coronary heart disease and stroke, by preventing the oxidation of cholesterol, blood clots and the build-up of cholesterol on the walls of blood vessels. Vitamin E also plays a role in preventing cancer. Vitamin E reduces the oxygen requirement of muscle, and thereby increases exercise capacity. It helps prevent the degeneration of nerve and muscle tissue. It may also aid post-surgical wound-healing and aid poor circulation, including varicose veins. The efficacy of vitamin E is enhanced by the mineral selenium and by vitamin C.

Deep frying, freezing, solvent extraction of edible oils, and commercial processing of food reduce their vitamin E content.

Good food sources are: wheatgerm oil, rapeseed oil, raw sunflower seeds, almonds, peanut butter and soya oil.

MINERALS

Minerals perform two functions: they form the solid parts of bones and teeth, and they take part in the biochemical processes of life. That is why a healthy mineral balance is a vital part of well-being.

Sound bones and teeth need a constant supply of minerals from the diet. Not surprisingly, many people think of bones and teeth as hard, static or even dead structures, but they are not. The parts of teeth beneath the gum and the hard, outside enamel is very much alive. So is bone. Bone is made up of a protein matrix containing blood vessels and small islands of cells. Deposits of calcium, magnesium and phosphorus form within this matrix. The highly specialised cells found in bone constantly break down and then rebuild these hard mineral deposits, creating a continual demand for new supplies.

Sixteen minerals have been identified as being necessary for life. Together, they form between 3 and 4% of the total body weight. Four minerals – calcium, magnesium, potassium and sodium are required in relatively large amounts, and are known as macronutrients. The other twelve essential minerals are needed in smaller amounts, and are called micronutrients; of this group, some – like selenium – are needed in such small amounts that they are known as 'trace' minerals.

The body normally contains minerals not used in normal life processes. They vary in their toxicity. It has been suggested that aluminium may be linked with Alzheimer's disease, but there is no scientific proof of this. Lead, on the other hand, which can be ingested in food, or absorbed through the lungs from petrol fumes, has been linked with learning difficulties and behavioural changes. Mercury is also very poisonous, harming the brain and nervous system, kidneys, and gut.

NUTRITIONAL THERAPY

For good health, minerals need to be kept in balance. Too little of one – magnesium, for example, can affect the way another mineral – calcium, in this case – functions. Correcting your mineral balance is a problem that is best addressed with specialist help.

MACROMINERALS

Calcium: The most abundant mineral in the human body, calcium is found in bone and soft tissue. It is needed for bones and teeth, blood-clotting and nerve and muscle function. Its levels are closely tied to the amount of vitamin D available. Calcium deficiency may aggravate allergies.

Food sources: dairy products and dark green leafy vegetables.

LEFT DAIRY PRODUCTS SUCH AS COTTAGE CHEESE ARE A GOOD SOURCE OF CALCIUM.

Magnesium: an intrinsic part of calcium metabolism. Most is found in bones, where, with calcium and phosphorus, it gives structure and strength. It is also essential for energy release, needed for DNA and RNA formation, and aids the normal function of muscle and nerves. Deficiency may be widespread in Western countries: symptoms include anxiety, insomnia, low blood sugar, and muscle twitches and cramps.

Food sources: peanuts, wholegrain products, white fish.

RIGHT WHOLEGRAIN PRODUCTS SUCH AS BROWN BREAD ARE VALUABLE SOURCES OF MINERALS SUCH AS MAGNESIUM AND PHOSPHORUS.

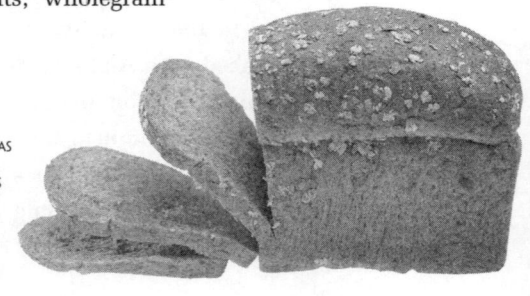

Phosphorus: Along with calcium, phosphorus is the major mineral component in bone and teeth. About 15 per cent is found in soft tissues, where it helps maintain the acid/alkaline balance of the body.
Food sources: wholegrain cereals, meat and dairy products.

Sodium: Sodium is a major component of all body fluids and, with potassium, is largely responsible for controlling the total water content in your body. It also plays a role in muscle and nerve function. Normally, excessive amounts of sodium ingested in food is excreted by the kidneys; however, when this fails, fluid is retained in the body, and causes swollen ankles and high blood pressure. In severe cases, this can lead to kidney failure, heart failure, and stroke. Deficiency is rare, but extensive sodium loss through sweat can cause muscle cramps and dehydration.

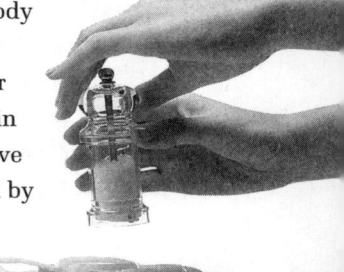

ABOVE PEOPLE WITH HIGH BLOOD PRESSURE AND KIDNEY DISEASE SHOULD AVOID ADDING SALT TO THEIR FOOD.

Food sources: most foods contain sodium. Excessive use of table salt (sodium chloride) can be dangerous for those suffering from high blood pressure or kidney disease.

TRACE MINERALS
Boron: This trace mineral is thought to play a role in controlling bone density. Food sources include soya, prunes and raisins.

Chromium: an essential part of glucose metabolism and control of blood fat levels. Deficiency results in poor glucose tolerance and high blood cholesterol levels. May increase lean muscle mass.
Food sources: egg yolk, molasses, beef.

Copper: essential for normal circulation, red blood cell formation, fatty acids oxidation, energy release, skin pigment formation, and brain function. Copper has antioxidant properties by itself, but as a constituent of the enzyme superoxide dismutase (S.O.D.) it becomes part of the body's natural system of antioxidant molecules. Copper deficiency, particularly when accompanied by selenium deficiency, increases the risk of heart disease. A high intake of zinc increases the need for copper.

Food sources: oysters, liver, yeast, olives and hazelnuts.

Iodine: Iodine is a necessary part of the hormones thyroxine and triiodothyronine, which control the metabolic rate of the body and maintain the integrity of connective tissue. Iodine deficiency causes 'goitre', a marked swelling in front of the neck; it may also result in cretinism in children. Worldwide, iodine deficiency causes more cases of preventable mental retardation than any other single factor.

Food sources of iodine include: kelp (seaweed), sea food.

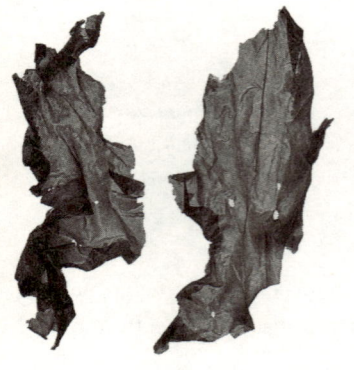

ABOVE KELP (SEAWEED) IS AN EXCELLENT SOURCE OF IODINE, IMPORTANT FOR REGULATING THE BODY'S METABOLISM.

Iron: Iron is an important part of the haemoglobin molecule in red blood cells that carries oxygen around the body. Iron is also found in muscle tissue, and aids in the release of energy from food. Women suffering high menstrual blood loss, vegetarians, pregnant women, athletes and older people may need iron supplements. Recent studies show that a surprising number of children are iron deficient.

Food sources: meat, bread and cereals, potatoes.

Manganese: This trace element is essential for growth and reproduction. It is an important part of the body's natural antioxidant system, and thereby helps prevent degenerative illnesses such as arthritis, coronary heart disease and cancer. It also promotes nerve function, healthy bones, synthesis of joint lubricant, and the formation of glycogen in the liver.

Food sources: tea, wholegrains, avocados and nuts.

Molybdenum: a trace element necessary for normal sexual function in men. Also needed for production of uric acid (a waste product) and iron metabolism. Molybdenum deficiency is thought to increase the risk of dental caries.

Food sources: Widespread in food including liver, wholegrains and pulses, sunflower seeds.

Potassium: This element is essential for muscle and nerve activity. It also plays a part in maintaining the acid/alkaline balance of the body. Deficiency can cause mental confusion, muscle weakness and abnormal heart beats. Causes for deficiency include the use of certain diuretics, the loss of body minerals through profuse sweating, and possibly the long-term use of certain antibiotics.

Food sources: fruit and vegetables.

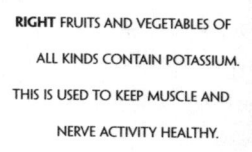

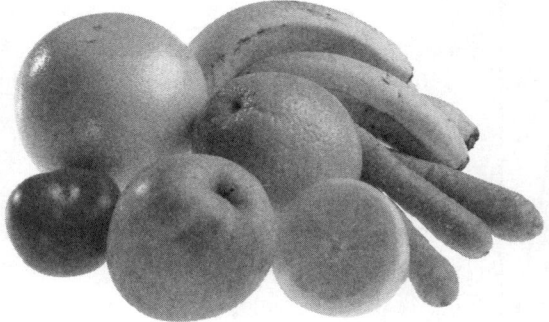

RIGHT FRUITS AND VEGETABLES OF ALL KINDS CONTAIN POTASSIUM. THIS IS USED TO KEEP MUSCLE AND NERVE ACTIVITY HEALTHY.

Selenium: This trace element facilitates the work of vitamins C and E. Plants gain their selenium content from the soil in which they are grown. Selenium forms part of the antioxidant molecule glutathione peroxidase. Selenium helps maintain the heart, helps produce thyroid hormone, promotes normal liver function, inhibits the action

NUTRITIONAL THERAPY

of toxic heavy metals, including mercury and lead. Parts of the world have low selenium soil levels, and therefore foods grown in these areas do not provide adequate quantities for good health.

Food sources: organ meats, shellfish, Brazil nuts, wholegrain food.

LEFT BRAZIL NUTS ARE AN EXCELLENT SOURCE OF SELENIUM, WHICH IS IMPORTANT FOR MAINTAINING THE HEALTH OF THE HEART.

ANTIOXIDANTS

I once asked a renowned American nutritionist what he thought was the most exciting aspect of modern nutrition. I had imagined he would mention enzymes, or perhaps the importance of the interaction between nutrition and genetics. 'Antioxidants' was his reply. 'These are the natural substances that hold the answer to major health problems suffered in Western societies'. A hundred years ago, most people died of acute conditions such as infections and accidents. Today, in Westernized cultures, most of us die of chronic illnesses such as cancer and heart disease. However, it is possible to see a time – not too far in the future – when this sad fact is altered by applying our growing knowledge of antioxidants.

Antioxidants in food are vitally important because they neutralize the damaging effects of free radicals. Free radicals are unstable molecules that form during the normal chemical workings of the body: with amazing speed, long, chain-like molecules are split and reassembled, fat and sugar molecules are reduced to energy and waste products, and electrons are ripped by one molecule from another and transferred to another. The molecule remaining – bare of one electron – is a free radical. It is highly reactive; because its nature is to grab on to another molecule and snatch away one of its electrons to satisfy its own imbalance, a free radical exists for a very short period of time.

As explained above, free radicals are created during normal biological processes. However, they are also created in large quantities under artificial conditions. In these cases, free radicals can do considerable damage to the community of molecules in which they were created and consequently to the body's cells and tissues.

Free radicals can form in response to smoking, stress (including excessive amounts of exercise), infection, radiation (including x-rays and sunlight), certain chemicals and environmental pollution from, for example, exhaust fumes. In other words, our modern lifestyle and environment subject us to higher levels of free radicals than any humans have faced before. Excessive amounts of free radicals can be a factor in disease. By damaging delicate fats and proteins in your body, free radicals may significantly increase risk of cancer, heart disease, degenerative diseases of the bone, and wrinkled skin.

The process by which electrons are whipped away from one molecule by another involves oxygen atoms, and for that reason is called 'oxidation'. Antioxidants are a valuable part of our daily diet because they are molecules that mop up the extra free radicals, and prevent them from doing damage.

The most important antioxidants are: vitamin C; vitamin E; beta-carotene (which the body uses to form vitamin A); a substance called 'reduced glutathione'; and three minerals –

selenium, zinc and molybdenum. There is no one food that is rich in all these nutrients. Vitamin C, for example, is a water-soluble compound found in watery parts of foods, like spinach leaves. Vitamin E is soluble in fats, and is found most abundantly in the oily substance of nuts and seeds. These antioxidant nutrients work together to protect your body, and you must eat a range of fruits, vegetables, nuts and seeds to obtain an adequate level.

LEFT NUTS, FRUITS AND VEGETABLES ALL HAVE IMPORTANT ANTIOXIDANT PROPERTIES.

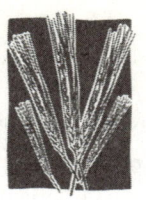

MIRACLES FROM PLANTS

CHAPTER SIX

The world of plants offers healing substances to help sustain well-being. From the dawn of human existence, healers have used herbs, berries, roots and leaves to bind wounds and fight fevers. Natural antibacterial and antiviral substances from nature were all they had to fight life-threatening illnesses. Now, through advances in modern science, the specific healing substances in plants can be identified and reproduced to use as medicines.

Scientists are searching the forests of the world looking for new compounds to treat disease. You, meanwhile, can take advantage of a miraculous storehouse of healing substances merely by increasing the variety and quantity of fruits and vegetables that you eat each day.

PLANTS THAT HEAL

The following is a short list of edible plants not mentioned above that are known to contain healing substances. The benefits of plants are only summarised here. If this subject interests you, there are excellent resource materials now available; some are listed under Further Reading (see pp.119–120).

ALGAE

An unusual food that may be a major future source of nourishment. Algae are organisms living on the divide between plant and animal life. Micro-algae, such as chlorella, spirulina and blue-green algae are rich in chlorophyll (the green substance in plants needed to combine carbon dioxide and water with energy from the sun to produce carbohydrates). These algae and are believed to help regulate the menstrual cycle, regulate calcium metabolism, and act as an anti-inflammatory. They also contain sulphur-rich lipids thought to have potential use in controlling AIDS. These ancient organisms are good sources of many required nutrients, including protein, beta-carotene, omega 3 and/or GLA fatty acids, and vitamin B12. The 'macro' algae – kombu, nori and wakame seaweed – also contain less significant amounts of B12.

ALFALFA SPROUTS

Used to treat breast-feeding problems and symptoms of endometriosis and the menopause. Alfalfa sprouts contain required nutrients as well as bioflavins, chlorophyll and enzymes that help break down protein. Detoxifies the body and benefits the urinary tract.

Warning: Alfalfa contains canavanine, a substance that may worsen rheumatoid arthritis and lupus erythematosus – an incurable inflammatory disease of connective tissue.

ALLIUM (GARLIC, ONION, LEEKS)

Antibacterial and antiviral substances in this family of foods may help control infection. Of value to those with weakened immune systems.

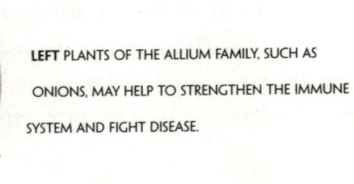

LEFT PLANTS OF THE ALLIUM FAMILY, SUCH AS ONIONS, MAY HELP TO STRENGTHEN THE IMMUNE SYSTEM AND FIGHT DISEASE.

ALOE VERA

Not a common edible plant, but one with such healing potential it is worth mentioning here. The juice from the leaves of this succulent are said to greatly benefit wound-healing, and to contain useful amino acids and minerals.

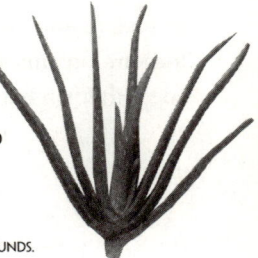

RIGHT JUICE FROM ALOE VERA LEAVES CAN SPEED THE HEALING OF WOUNDS.

ANISE

Anise is the seed of a liquorice-flavoured herb. It is used in various ways to treat asthma, bad breath, sore throat and colds. It is also said to help remove sexual inhibition in women and help erectile problems in men.

BLUEBERRIES (AND CRANBERRIES)

Contain arbutin, which acts as a diuretic and natural antibiotic.

CARROTS

Well known for the beta-carotene that they contain (the pre-cursor of vitamin A needed to prevent night-blindness), carrots are also said to contain compounds that help to lower blood pressure.

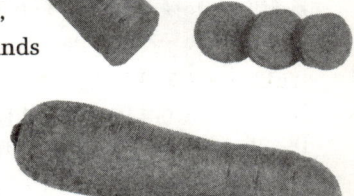

RIGHT CARROTS ARE RICH IN ANTIOXIDANTS, THE MOST SIGNIFICANT OF WHICH IS BETA-CAROTENE.

CRANBERRIES

Useful for controlling bladder infections. A substance within the fruit changes the physical form of potentially harmful bacteria so that they can no longer cling to the walls of the bladder and establish colonies of infection.

DILL

An ancient and effective aid to digestion.

Caution: do not use consume more than one tablespoon of the chopped, fresh herb per day.

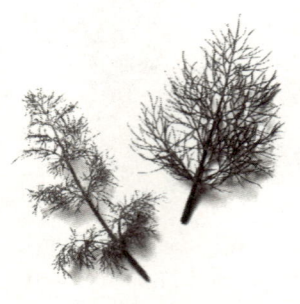

FENNEL

Fennel is a herb that grows wild, and is used in several healing systems. In Traditional Chinese Medicine, it is used to treat indigestion, gastroenteritis and abdominal pain. Fennel has been used in Ayurvedic pharmacology for more than a thousand years with much the same purpose. It is also prized as part of the masalas – or traditional blends of culinary spice mix – and chewed to freshen the breath after a meal. The essential oil of fennel is sometimes used in aromatherapy to promote the flow of breast milk. Modern nutritionists value fennel seeds as a source of minerals and B-vitamins.

ABOVE FENNEL IS A HERB THAT IS OFTEN USED TO TREAT DIGESTIVE PROBLEMS. IT ALSO CONTAINS VALUABLE NUTRIENTS.

GRAPES

A popular bit of modern health lore claims that red wine – drunk in moderation – contains compounds (phenols) believed to protect the body from a dangerous build-up of cholesterol. Red wine is red because of pigments under the skins of the red grapes from which it is made. Similar substances are found in garlic, onions, blueberries, bilberries and blackberries.

RIGHT GRAPES CONTAIN COMPOUNDS THAT HELP TO PREVENT THE BUILD-UP OF CHOLESTEROL

GREEN TEA

Rich in natural antioxidants, antibacterial and antiviral substances, green tea is thought to help lower the risk of cancer and heart disease, improve dental health, fight flu and other viral infections, and reduce blood cholesterol levels. Scientists in Great Britain have found that four to five cups of green tea a day might help reduce blood pressure and lower cholesterol levels.

TOMATOES

Tomatoes contain a group of molecules called lycopenes, pigments that are found in highest concentrations in cells just under the skin, have been found to be powerful antioxidants. There is reason to hope that they will help in the fight against both heart disease and prostate cancer. As these are most available to us in tomatoes that have been cooked, good sources are tomato purée, pasta sauce and tomato catsup.

OLIVE OIL

Virgin (unrefined) olive oil has been recognised as being useful in the prevention of heart disease. It is also useful in the control of gallbladder and liver conditions. A combination therapy using digestive enzymes and herbs, substituting low-fat protein for high-fat red meat, and including an increased intake of olive oil and nuts can be very effective. This is the type of treatment that should be undertaken with the help of a trained professional.

RIGHT COOKING WITH VIRGIN OLIVE OIL IS A SIMPLE AND DELICIOUS WAY OF HELPING TO PROTECT THE HEALTH OF YOUR HEART.

PARSLEY

A useful diuretic that also helps to control bladder infections.

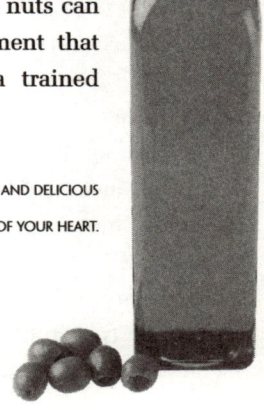

PINEAPPLE

Contains compounds believed to aid bruising, carpal tunnel syndrome, gout, heartburn, skin problems and stomach ulcers. Pineapple is also thought to be useful in weight control. Certainly this is a fruit that should appear on your menu at least once a week.

SOYA BEANS

We now know that soya beans are not just an important plant source of good protein – they contain compounds shown to be effective in fighting cancer and heart disease. The anti-cancer compounds contained in this rather bland-tasting little bean include: insoflavones (compounds similar to oestrogen that may help prevent hormone-dependent cancers of the breast and prostate); genistein (a substance that seems to block the spread of cancer cells); daidzein and daidzin; which appear to block the growth of new blood vessels needed by developing tumours; and phytic acids (shown to slow or stop the growth of tumours in animal studies). Every month, at least two studies appear in the international medical press that takes us a step closer to fully understanding the healing and preventive potential of this basic food.

LEFT SOYA BEANS ARE EXTREMELY NUTRITIOUS AND CONTAIN NUMEROUS ANTICANCER COMPOUNDS.

WILD YAM

Compounds similar to oestrogen found in this plant are said to make it a useful means of treating a number of problems women suffer, including breast pain during nursing and symptoms of the menopause.

From these few examples, you can see that the inquiry into phytochemicals and their potential as protective and healing agents is one of the most exciting aspects of modern health care. But, does this research belong to the discipline of medicine? Or to the increasingly important field of nutritional therapy? Perhaps it is here, in this rapidly growing area of scientific investigation, that nutritional therapy will develop its most dynamic aspect, and regain the scientific prominence the study of nutrition lost five decades ago.

Non-Food Healing Plants

Taking advantage of new findings, a number of plant products are now available from supermarkets and health food stores to meet increasing public demand. These products blur the boundary between nutrition and herbal medicine. All of these are used in nutritional therapy, and may be taken in combination with concentrates of purified nutrients and healing food plants to treat particular health conditions. Notice that most of the plants I mention below are not used as food. The number of these new products on the market is bewildering. Frequently used plant products include:

Echinacea, used to strengthen the immune system, fight bacterial and viral infections, and help some cases of chronic fatigue syndrome.

Ginkgo Biloba, to aid memory (this plant extract has shown some promise in the treatment of the early stages of Alzheimer's disease).

Lecithin, not a plant but a component extracted from soya beans that aids liver problems, including gallstones, and contains substances important for normal brain function.

Milk Thistle, used in the treatment of psoriasis, liver problems and gallstones.

Psyllium, a plant used to aid constipation;

St. John's Wort, a natural anti-depressant. This plant extract does not affect behaviour as

ABOVE ECHINACEA TINCTURE HELPS TO BOOST THE IMMUNE SYSTEM.

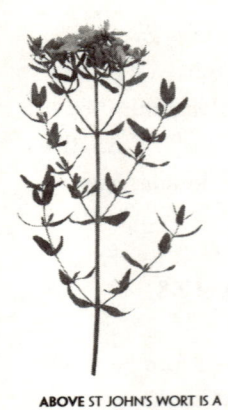

NUTRITIONAL THERAPY

quickly as some pharmaceutical antidepressants, but appears to have fewer side effect.

All of these products should be treated with respect. People can have reactions to anything. Just because something is 'natural' does not mean it is always safe. If you think any plant or supplement is causing side-effects, such as dizziness or headache, stop taking it at once.

ABOVE ST JOHN'S WORT IS A NATURAL ANTIDEPRESSANT.

CANCER-FIGHTING FOODS

There are a number of substances in certain foods that are believed to fight cancer. Different compounds combat cancer in different ways. For example, a major component of citrus oils, d-limonene, has been found to inhibit cancer-causing chemicals. Plants of the cruciferous family, which include brassica such as cabbage and broccoli, are rich sources of groups of compounds known as indoles, phenols and aromatic isothiocyanates, which have all been shown to inhibit the transformation of normal cells into cancer cells.

Research has shown that certain mushrooms have powerful anticancer properties: Japanese shiitake mushrooms are an example.

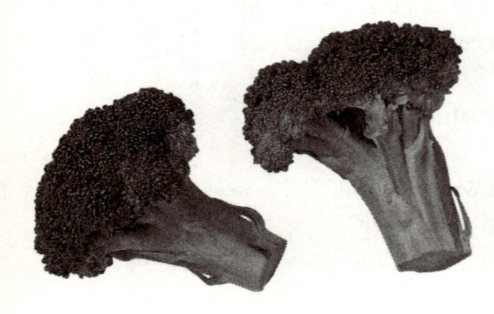

LEFT BROCCOLI AND OTHER CRUCIFEROUS VEGETABLES ARE VALUABLE ANTI-CANCER FOODS.

A water extract of fruit bodies from the very costly and rare matsutake mushroom (called 'King of Mushrooms' in Japan) has been shown to boost the immune system and selectively kill cancer cells caused by viral infection. The study of the protective and curative properties of these mushrooms holds great promise, not only in the fight against cancer, but also to help against diseases involving the immune system, such as AIDS.

HERBS AND SPICES

Common spices and herbs contain powerful compounds that fight infection. James A. Duke, Ph.D., author of The Green Pharmacy, found in a study that coriander and liquorice contained 20 natural antibacterial substances, while oregano contained 19, ginger 15, black pepper 14, garlic 13, cinnamon and cumin 11, and bay leaf 10. By dry weight, thyme is said to contain up to 21.3 per cent bactericidal compounds. No wonder that it has been used for centuries as a flavouring in meat dishes that could spoil. It is noticeable that most great cuisines in the world have their own identifying formulation of herbs and spices. Italian food is full of garlic, basil, parsley and oregano. Food from the Indian sub-continent brings to your table the colour and aroma of turmeric, cardamom, mustard and – again – garlic. All these wonderful ingredients give more than interest to the dishes in which they are prepared; they bring nutrition. Parsley is a rich source of vitamins, minerals, and like all green leafy plants, the important phytochemical chlorophyll. Turmeric is full of minerals and curcumin, a natural compound with anti-cancer properties. So, when you plan variety in your food, make sure you also include a variety of spices and herbs. You will be well rewarded for it.

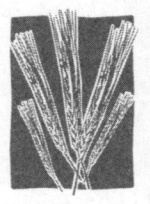

FOOD SUPPLEMENTS

CHAPTER SEVEN

*S*upplements are no substitute for eating a balanced diet, but they can have a powerful influence on your health. This chapter provides general information about the selection and use of food supplements. It is a guide, and not meant to be all-inclusive, or provide all the information required to treat specific ailments. Readers are always advised to seek help from a trained professional before undertaking any course of therapy.

There are several reasons why food supplements can be useful. Modern living places strains on your body and therefore increases its need for specific nutrients. Supplements 'top up' the amounts of nutrients you ingest in food, to provide an adequate supply for normal biological activity in your body. In addition, certain nutrients have powerful curative effects when consumed in amounts larger than those available in a normal diet. Vitamin B6, for example, has been shown to help alleviate symptoms of premenstrual syndrome when consumed in levels in excess of those recommended for normal human health.

RIGHT SUPPLEMENTS CAN HELP TO TOP UP THE VITAMINS AND MINERALS THAT YOUR BODY REQUIRES.

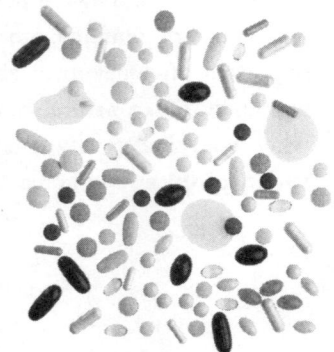

Forms of Supplements

Supplements come in many different forms. Among the most popular available are:

- Multivitamins – these are compounded blends of vitamins and minerals, balanced to reflect expert opinion on average human nutritional requirements. Contents vary widely, and it is important to read labels and see exactly which nutrients have been included.
- Multiminerals - combinations of essential minerals combined in quantities greater than those usually found in multivitamin products.
- Single nutrient supplements. These may contain individual vitamins (vitamin B6, for example), or a mineral, such as iron. Amino acids are also sold in isolation.
- Evening primrose oil and star flower oil, which contain a high amount of the essential fatty acid known as GLA.
- Fish oil, for its high content of the fatty acids EPA and DHA, which have been shown to protect the heart.
- Zinc and vitamin C, to help the immune system, fight infection, promote wound-healing and energy balance.
- Vitamin C tables, to boost the immune system.
- Vitamins A, C and E, together with the mineral selenium – a powerful antioxidant blend that helps fight ageing, cancer and heart disease, and combat problems of arthritis and painful joints.
- Folic acid, a member of the B-vitamin family taken by women during early pregnancy to support the development of foetal brain and neuronal tissue.
- Calcium and magnesium, which help to build strong bones and teeth and prevent osteoporosis.

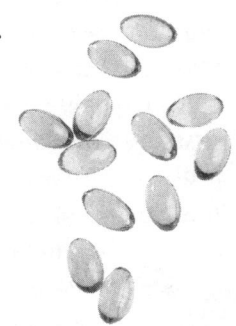

ABOVE EVENING PRIMROSE OIL SUPPLEMENTS ARE A VALUABLE SOURCE OF ESSENTIAL FATTY ACIDS.

Buying Supplements

For the untrained person, selecting which supplement to buy can be very complicated. It is useful to consult an expert on which product meets your requirements. Several of the major manufacturers of vitamin products have excellent telephone help lines. Alternatively, you could consult an in-store advisor in your local health food shop or chemist. Talk to experts from several companies before making a choice. A nutritional therapist will also give advice on what products are appropriate for you.

Food supplements are available in tablet, powder and capsule form. They vary in both the substances they contain and their amounts. Do not buy a product on the basis of price alone. Always read the label before buying to confirm that a product contains what you want in the quantities you need. Some inexpensive products claim to provide all your daily requirements for vitamins and minerals, but on inspection are seen to contain very modest amounts of nutrients.

Always buy from a reputable firm, and accept that there are no cheap substitutes for quality. An inexpensive product may contain the nutrients you want, but not in their most natural form. For example, seed oils – flaxseed, evening primrose and star flower (borage) – can be extracted in several ways. The least costly method is to simply grind and press the seed pulp. However, considerable heat is generated during this process, which damages the valuable essential fatty acids in these seeds. Another method of extraction involves crushing seeds and extracting the oils with solvents. Little heat is generated during this process, and it is safe because the solvents used are highly volatile, and easily removed from the final product. Buy vitamin E in gelatine capsules; vitamin E is fat-soluble, and changing it into a dry, solid form requires a change in its structure.

LEFT VITAMIN E IS BEST PURCHASED IN GELATINE CAPSULES.

Store vitamins in a cool, dark place. Oily supplements should be stored in the refrigerator once their package is opened. Some nutrients are synergistic and should therefore be taken together; for example, calcium and vitamin D.

Cautions with Supplements

When taking supplements, there are several things that you need to be cautious about. If you take two or more diet supplements during a day, make sure you are not overdosing on any one nutrient. It may take time, but sit down and write a list of all the nutrients in the supplements you take, and add up the contents from each supplement. Remember, these combine with nutrients in your diet, so the total amount you consume is the sum of your supplements and food intake.

A number of other cautions are:
- Vitamin A, if taken in excess over time, can be toxic because it builds up in the liver and is not eliminated. Beta-carotene, which the body converts into vitamin A, is a safe alternative, because once the body has enough it tends to slow down the conversion process.
- Vitamin A should not be taken with drugs derived from vitamin A that are used to treat acne.
- People with kidney stones should not take more than one gram of vitamin C per day.
- Very large quantities of vitamin D – in the region of 1000 mcg a day – may be harmful.
- A very high intake of copper, iodine, iron, molybdenum, selenium and zinc can be toxic (see table for safe doses).
- Massive doses of niacin (of three to six grams a day) may cause liver changes. However, this is an excessive amount.

ABOVE VITAMIN A SHOULD NOT BE TAKEN FOR EXTENDED PERIODS.

NUTRITIONAL THERAPY

- Vitamin B6 may cause sensory changes, such as tingling and numbness of the fingers and toes, when taken in very high quantities over a long period of time (two to seven grams a day). Stick to lower quantities.
- If you have problems with stomach acidity, or ulcers, take only a buffered form of vitamin C.
- Supplements containing beta-carotene have been hailed as a highly effective antioxidant. However, some doubt has been cast on their safety because a study involving a large number of people suggested that beta-carotene contributed to the risk of lung cancer in smokers. If you smoke, boost your antioxidant levels with other antioxidant vitamins, and natural substances such as lycopene (see p.69). Better still, enjoy a diet rich in red and yellow fruits and vegetables. These are good sources of natural beta-carotene.

A golden rule is to avoid taking excessive amounts of any nutrient. Supplements should also be treated with caution because of the chance that they could interact with nutrients. Nutrients are active ingredients in the biology of the human body. Their behaviour can be affected by a deficiency or surplus of other nutrients, and with prescribed medications. Always check with your chemist or nutritionist when you begin a new drug therapy or alter your intake of nutrients. A few examples of interactions are:

- Riboflavin is unstable in the presence of the antibiotics tetracycline and erythromycin, and should therefore be taken at different times.
- Vitamin B6 should not be taken with certain anticonvulsant drugs: always check with your nutritionist, chemist or doctor.
- People with insulin-dependent diabetes should seek advice before increasing their intake of the mineral chromium.

LEFT RIBOFLAVIN SHOULD NOT BE TAKEN WITH CERTAIN ANTIBIOTICS.

- Certain diuretics and cortisone may increase excretion of zinc, justifying an increased intake of this important mineral, while staying well within safe limits.

If you are uncertain, it is always wise to take food supplements and pharmaceutical medicines at different times.

UPPER SAFE LEVEL FOR DAILY SELF-SUPPLEMENTATION

[Information supplied by Quest Vitamins Professional Product Manual. Although these are figures from one source, they are generally accepted values.]

MICRONUTRIENT	UNIT	UPPER SAFE LEVEL
Vitamin A	mcg	2300
Vitamin D	mcg	10
Vitamin E	mg	800
Beta-carotene	mg	20
Thiamin [B1]	mg	100
Riboflavin [B2]	mg	200
Niacin amide [B3]	mg	450
acid	mg	150
Pyridoxine [B6]	mg	200
Folic Acid [B complex]	mcg	400
Cobalamin [B12]	mcg	500
Biotin [B complex]	mcg	500
Pantothenic acid [B complex]	mg	500
Vitamin C	mg	2000
Calcium	mg	1500
Phosphorus	mg	1500

Magnesium	mg	350
Copper	mg	5
Chromium	mcg	200
Iodine	mcg	500
Iron	mg	15
Manganese	mg	15
Molybdenum	mcg	200
Selenium	mcg	200
Zinc	mg	15

Note: 1g (gram) = 1000 mg; 1 mg (milligram) = 1000 mcg (micrograms)

Case Study

Victoria suffered from pre-menstrual tension [PMT] and heavy periods that made her moody and sluggish at work. Her moods also affected her social life, and added to her problems at home. Frustration and self-pity meant that the biscuit jar was usually close at hand when she watched television in the evenings, and as she often bought a take-away on her way home from work, she ate burgers and chips at least four times a week.

An infected cut on her right foot caused Victoria to visit her family doctor, who was surprised by her general appearance: round-shouldered, overweight and pale. When asked how she felt, Victoria blurted out her feeling about how PMT was affecting her job, and asked for medication. Instead, Victoria's doctor asked her to make an appointment to see the clinic's nutritional therapist. At first she resisted, thinking that she would just receive a patronising diet sheet. However, the nutritional therapist gave her a comprehensive interview, asked her to complete a lengthy questionnaire, and took some blood and urine samples. When all the results had been studied, a course of treatment was agreed upon. Victoria's treatment consisted of high-quality multivitamin and mineral tablets, Evening Primrose Oil, a vitamin B6 supplement, and a sheet of facts describing food substitutes she might try: tofu and low-fat cheese sandwiches instead of burgers and chips, and snacking on popcorn instead of biscuits, for example. Finally, the nutritional therapist gave Victoria some advice: the person to whom she should be most kind in the world was herself. Black moods ultimately hurt her more than anyone else and she had the right to be good to herself.

Victoria began taking the supplements prescribed, and noticed a difference in her energy level and general well-being within a month. Her PMT improved over the next two months, and she found she had energy to start exercising after work. Six months later, she looked in the mirror and saw a far healthier and happier person.

Case Study

Meryl was a young mother with a six-month-old baby. She constantly felt exhausted. A friend suggested that she talk to her doctor, but Meryl insisted that things would improve. Over the next few weeks, she began suffering one minor skin or gum infection after another, and decided to ask her doctor to give her a prescription for antibiotics. While she was at the surgery, the doctor took some blood samples to check Meryl's blood cells, and suggested that she talk to the clinic nutritionist. The tests showed that Meryl had a low haemoglobin level, and was probably not

NUTRITIONAL THERAPY

getting enough iron in her diet. A vitamin and mineral supplement, rich in iron, was prescribed. Working with the nutritionist, Meryl learned how to use the tablets for maximum benefit. The nutritionist also explained how to increase the level of iron in Meryl's diet by eating more lean meat, dark green leafy vegetables, and sardines. After a few months, Meryl's blood haemoglobin level was normal, and she no longer required iron supplements. Better still, she had energy and no longer suffered from irritating infections.

Wanting a strong and healthy baby, Meryl took excellent care of herself during her pregnancy. But once the baby was born, she did not pay the same attention to what she ate. The constant attention needed by her baby, and the new housekeeping chores that his presence created, took more time than she expected. As a result, she drifted into the habit of having a piece of toast and tea for breakfast, a handful of biscuits and a cola drink for lunch, and easy-to-prepare processed foods for dinner with her husband. As a result, Meryl's intake of necessary nutrients was thrown off balance. The monitored use of dietary supplements and reintroduction of sensible food choices restored her to health.

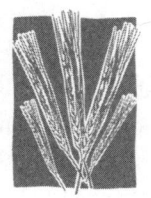

SELF-HELP AND DISEASE PREVENTION

CHAPTER EIGHT

The links between nutrition and disease have been widely recognized. As the understanding of this relationship grows, our ability to effectively prevent many illnesses, both major and minor, improves. This fact is especially important in affluent Westernized countries, where environmental pollution and poor eating habits dominated by the consumption of processed foods undermine the natural body processes that fight disease.

CHEMICAL THREATS IN THE MODERN WORLD

The man-made chemicals in cosmetics, cleaning products, and artificial enhancers used in foods are pervasive in the modern world. In addition, modern methods of growing food often involve the use of organophosphate pesticides and fertilizers, which are so dangerous

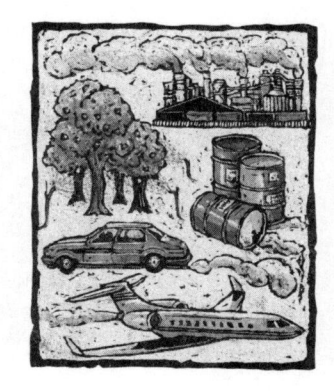

RIGHT PEOPLE IN THE MODERN WORLD FACE AN UNPRECEDENTED HEALTH THREAT FROM ENVIRONMENTAL POLLUTION.

that they are closely related to deadly nerve gases. All these chemicals have no normal place in the cells and tissues of the human body, but they find their way there. Each of these non-natural chemicals was tested and approved before it was allowed to be sold on the market. However, man-made chemicals are usually tested individually for safety. How they behave after becoming part of the 'cocktail' of man-made chemicals that build up in our bodies is impossible to test. Each person's life experience is unique, and so each has been exposed to a unique combination of chemicals. Detoxifying these chemicals and finding ways to cope with their abnormal presence as they mix with normal nutrients are two of the greatest concerns of nutritional therapy. Our best defence is a healthy diet that includes foods that help detoxify our tissues (see p.33, detoxification diets).

MODERN DIETS AND FOOD PRODUCTION

Through modern technology, farmers are producing more food, and manufacturers are providing a wider variety of foods than ever before. Nonetheless, the number of people suffering from diseases thought to have roots in underlying nutritional deficiencies is increasing. Why is this? We in the West are anything but under-fed. Some experts argue that we are over-fed and over-nourished. But this is not true. Stripping out vital nutrients through modern methods of food technology, plus our poor eating habits, help to make us over-fed and under-nourished.

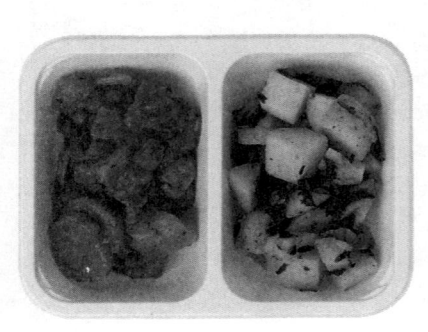

LEFT MODERN FOOD PRODUCTION METHODS MEAN THAT MANY OF THE MEALS WE EAT ARE RELATIVELY LOW IN NUTRIENTS.

Unfortunately, the foods that most of us enjoy eating are often those that are potentially damaging to our health. Where we once ate modest amounts of fats, on average we now ingest about 40 per cent of our calories from fats. According to World Health Organization experts, the typical caloric intake for young men should be about 25% of total calories: for women of childbearing age, the figure is around 30%. The excessive intake of fat that most of us eat encourages weight gain, over-stimulates certain metabolic processes, and reduces our desire to eat fruits, cereals and vegetables – the very foods that contain the nutrients required to combat the damaging effects of environmental pollution.

More damaging is the fact that most of the fat we eat is saturated animal fat: not the mono- and polyunsaturated fats known to be healthy for us (see pp.52–53). High dietary levels of saturated animal fats are statistically linked with cardiovascular illnesses and certain forms of cancer. Large stores of saturated fats in the body are believed to be damaging. One example of the reasons suggested for the possible link between fat and cancer is that fat cells produce oestrogen, and excessive oestrogen levels may help stimulate the growth of hormone-dependent tumours.

Our modern lifestyle also means we do not use, or burn off, calories in the same way, and so we tend to become obese. A hundred years ago, people were more physically active than most of us are today. They used up the calories they ingested by doing physical work and walking. Today, instead of walking we often drive to work. Our jobs are increasingly sedentary: more and more of us sit at desks or computer terminals all day – storing the calories we eat as fat instead of burning them off. We are also eating more fatty foods than people in the past. Extra fat crowds organs, adds to the pressure on leg joints, and encourages poor posture that can interfere with normal breathing. Increasing daily activity levels does more than burn off unwanted calories; physical exercise strengthens muscles, sinews and bones, and causes you to breathe deeply and increase your heart rate. Good eating habits and an informed choice of foods, combined with other components of a healthy lifestyle, can help to prevent many of the common illnesses suffered in modern society.

ILLNESS AND NUTRITIONAL DEFICIENCIES

Diseases caused by vitamin and mineral deficiencies have been recognized for centuries. James Lind in the 18th century discovered that a lack in vitamin C caused scurvy. In following years, it was discovered that the terrible symptoms of beriberi are completely reversed by foods containing vitamin B1 (thiamine). One form of beriberi causes severe water retention, and the other affects the nervous system, producing symptoms similar to that of serious mental illness. Pellagra, a potentially fatal disease with symptoms including diarrhoea and mental confusion, is caused by niacin deficiency and can be reversed if the sufferer eats foods rich in this vitamin. When severe deficiency diseases of this nature are treated with the appropriate nutrient, improvement in the patient's condition is often obvious within 24 hours.

There is increasing evidence that many diseases of modern society are caused by nutritional deficiencies. These are not the extreme nutritional deficiencies that result in conditions like scurvy and pellagra. Instead, these are long-term, borderline deficiencies caused when a person's diet contains too little of one or more

LEFT EATING A WELL-BALANCED DIET CAN HELP TO AVOID BOTH NUTRITIONAL DEFICIENCIES AND DEGENERATIVE DISEASES.

SELF-HELP AND DISEASE PREVENTION

nutrients to constantly maintain the body's normal biological processes. Over time this may lead to degenerative illnesses such as cardiovascular disease, arthritis, and some forms of cancer.

Deficiency diseases are difficult to treat because symptoms are rarely obvious as nutrient levels fall and tissues weaken. It is also the nature of a poor or inadequate diet to cause borderline deficiency in more than one nutrient at the same time. For example, if vegans do not obtain the full complement of essential amino acids that the body needs, enzymes and tissues dependant on specific amino acids can begin to fail. Also, unless vegans take vitamin supplements, or eat enriched foods, they risk suffering a vitamin B12 deficiency.

What can be done? The basic advice is the same for everyone: eat a balanced diet rich in a variety of fruits and vegetables, and containing a modest amount of fat. An increasing number of nutrition experts would also advise you to supplement your diet to suit your lifestyle.

STRENGTHENING THE IMMUNE SYSTEM

One of the best ways to prevent disease is to strengthen the immune system. The immune system is the collection of cells and substances in the body that identify and destroy potentially harmful material. This harmful material may be a colony of bacteria growing in a

RIGHT THE LYMPH SYSTEM IS THE HEART OF THE BODY'S IMMUNE SYSTEM, FIGHTING AGAINST DISEASE AND INFECTION.

wound, or tumour cells developing as part of a major organ. Tears, for example, not only wash away potentially harmful substances and organisms, but also produce lysozyme, an enzyme that destroys bacteria. This same enzyme also helps to protect the mouth. Mucus, a sticky substance produced in the respiratory system, captures bacteria, and, with the help of cilia (cells specially adapted with hairs) help sweep the invaders away or into the path of 'killer' cells (phagocytes), which engulf and destroy them. Your stomach, intestines and genito-urinary system contain harmless bacteria that help control the number of potentially harmful organisms. And the skin, the body's largest organ, provides a protective layer over the whole body.

A weakened immune system leaves the body vulnerable to attack from many factors. The immune system can be weakened by stress, lack of a properly balanced diet (especially one with a low intake of antioxidants), exposure to harmful chemicals, treatment with radiation or chemotherapy and exposure to environmental pollutants. By understanding the complex nature of the immune system, it is possible to gain some idea of the complex blend of raw materials – or nutrients – that it needs.

Foods important for strengthening the immune system include those rich in zinc, selenium, magnesium, vitamins B1, C and E, co-enzyme Q10, and essential fatty acids. Eat more protein-rich food, fruits and vegetables rich in vitamin C; red and orange fruits and vegetables for their antioxidant content; and wheatgerm, nuts and vegetable oils known as being good sources of vitamin E. Reducing your intake of processed carbohydrates and animal fats is essential. You should also consider cutting down on your consumption of alcohol and caffeine.

Supplements that aid the immune system include: garlic, leeks, onions and extracts of echinacea. If you have an infection, you should consume the red and black fruits (such as grapes, blueberries, cranberries and blackcurrants) that are known to be rich in natural antibacterial compounds.

SELF-HELP FOR SPECIFIC AILMENTS

What follows are suggestions as to how you can adapt your nutrient intake to best prevent or alleviate some of the common illnesses and ailments in modern life. Note, however, that professional advice is an important aspect of nutritional healing. If you feel you are gaining improvement by altering your diet but want faster results, or if you find no relief from the measures you take at home, seek help from an expert.

CARDIOVASCULAR DISEASE

About a third of a million people in Britain alone die of coronary heart disease (CHD) each year. Although we are doing much to treat the disease, it remains our number one killer. It was once thought to strike mainly middle-aged and older men, but an increasing number of women now suffer from high blood pressure, angina, high cholesterol levels, arteries blocked with fatty plaque, and blood clots in the blood vessels of heart.

There appears to be a genetic factor in the development of heart disease, and recent studies suggest that poor maternal diet during pregnancy increases the risk of high blood pressure. Despite these factors, there are ways to reduce risk. Proper exercise and reduced levels of stress help to prevent CHD, but a healthy diet is the most important form of protection. Free radicals play a significant role in CHD, making antioxidant-rich food and supplements containing antioxidants important. Also, as smoking and air pollution play a part in causing CHD, you are advised to stop smoking.

Nutritional therapists also advocate the following:
- Reduce your intake of saturated fats by substituting plant oils rich in monounsaturated and polyunsaturated fats.
- Enjoy foods high in soluble fibre, such as oats, lentils and beans, to help reduce the level of cholesterol in your body.
- Have a meal based on oily fish at least three times a week, or take fish oil supplements to increase your intake of omega-3 fatty acids.

- Select foods and supplements that balance your calcium and magnesium intake.
- Maintain a diet rich in GLA, an omega-6 fatty acid.
- Include co-enzyme Q10 in your diet to help strengthen heart muscle. (This is particularly important in the treatment of heart failure.)

You should begin your prevention programme now. Autopsies show that even very young people suffer degeneration of their cardiovascular tissues.

CANCER

The word 'cancer' is a general term covering a group of diseases with one shared characteristic: the run-away growth of abnormal cells. We hear most about cancers of the lungs, breasts, digestive system, blood, prostate and skin, but abnormal and spreading growth also occurs in the pancreas, liver and other organs. Unlike benign tumours, which stay contained in one place, cancerous growths move out of their original environment and expand to erode and destroy the tissues and nerves around them. Cells from the original growth can break away, and spread through the bloodstream to other sites, where they establish satellite tumours, called metastases. After heart disease, cancer is the biggest killer in the United Kingdom, with almost a quarter of a million new cases reported each year.

We tend to think of cancer as being a new disease, but it is not. It is common in fish and birds, farm and wild animals, and has been part of human suffering from the earliest days of our species. Despite the billions of dollars spent worldwide during the

LEFT CANCER IS ONE OF THE WORLD'S BIGGEST KILLERS AND HAS MANY POSSIBLE CAUSES.

RIGHT THERE IS A WELL ESTABLISHED LINK BETWEEN SMOKING AND THE DEVELOPMENT OF CANCER, PARTICULARLY LUNG CANCER.

past five decades on the causes of cancer, we are only a little more the wiser. We know that cancer has a genetic aspect: some of us have genes programmed for breast cancer, for example. We know that cigarette smoking causes cancer: cigarettes contain some of the most powerful carcinogens (cancer-causing agents) known to man. Hard scientific evidence indicates that certain naturally occurring substances in the foods we eat cause cancer. Probably the most dramatic example of this is liver cancer, one form of which is caused by a substance produced by a common mould that thrives on stored, damp grain and nuts. The carcinogen is called aflatoxin, and it causes many of the deaths from cancer in Africa. Links have been made between certain viruses and cancer. We are also aware that excessive exposure to ultra-violet radiation in sunlight, excessive alcohol intake, and a person's reproductive and sexual history play roles in the development of certain cancers, as do occupational hazards (like asbestos) and exposure to industrial pollution.

Specific cancers may have specific causes. Cancers of the bladder, cervix, mouth, oesophagus, pancreas and throat have all been linked to poor dietary levels of vitamin C, for example. A high intake of salty, smoked and pickled food has been linked with stomach cancer.

Folic acid appears to be important in the prevention of cervical cancer. Low levels are found in sufferers, and research suggests cervical cancer cell growth is slowed by increased levels of this vitamin. The risk of developing cancers of the breast, uterus, colon, prostate and rectum are reduced in populations enjoying a high-fibre diet.

Faced by the long list of causes of cancer, we must ask – how can we protect ourselves? There is little we can do about our genetic make-up. Responses to other causes are obvious, however: do not smoke, avoid excessive exposure to the sun, drink alcohol in moderation, and eat food from sources that you trust are pure and free from man-made or natural contamination. In addition to these methods, there is exciting news about the protective properties of substances in food. It may be that nutritional therapy will prove to be one of our most important weapons in the fight against cancer.

A growing body of scientific evidence suggests that the biological processes leading to the onset of cancer are slow and have several stages. Underlying nutritional deficiencies appear important early on, when the natural biological activities within a cell are disrupted. For this reason, a constant balanced flow of nutrients is important in cancer prevention.

It also appears that an increased intake of certain vitamins and minerals specifically reduces the risk of cancer by several means. For example, free radicals are known to damage delicate molecules that play essential roles in the structure of cells and their biological activity. This damage is thought to trigger abnormal cell division and replication, leading to the first stages of tumour growth. Antioxidant substances in foods – such as vitamins A, C and E, selenium and lycopene – block the action of free radicals and reduce this source of cancer risk. The practice of nutritional therapy takes advantage of this knowledge by prescribing foods and diet supplements rich in antioxidant vitamins and minerals. (Antioxidant foods are discussed on pp.62–64.)

Foods rich in phytochemicals also appear to reduce the risk of cancer. Isoflavones contained in soya, for example, hold great promise for the prevention and possible early treatment of hormone-dependant cancers, such as those of the breast and prostate. This effect probably partially explains the difference in cancer rates between women living in Japan and eating a traditional diet and women eating a Western diet.

Members of the Cruciferous plant family, such as broccoli, cabbage, kale, are known to contain many natural cancer-fighting compounds. You can gain the benefits of these plants by including them liberally in your diet – or by using plant preparations containing concentrates of these substances.

Nutritional therapy fights cancer in ways that combine the effects of diet and supplements to: build the underlying good health of normal tissue; strengthen the immune system to destroy emerging abnormal cells; block damaging free radicals; and suppress the growth of cancer cells once they have begun to multiply. Other mechanisms are yet to be discovered. For example, garlic appears to protect against stomach cancer, but we are not sure why. We are a long way from identifying all the cancer-fighting substances in plants, but the search has proven to hold great promise.

CANDIDIASIS AND THRUSH
Reduce the amount of red meat and dairy products you eat: enjoy fish and vegetable protein foods instead. Several glasses of cranberry juice a day will help to control associated bladder problems.

CATARRH
For the occasional bout of catarrh, eat spicy Asian foods, garlic and chilli peppers. If the condition persists, try eliminating all cows' milk products from your diet. Substitute ewe and sheep's milk or soya products. Many people experience remarkable relief from symptoms in a matter of a few days.

CONSTIPATION
Include a pot of live soya yoghurt in your diet each day. Increase your intake of high-fibre foods – including pulses and grains – so that they become a standard part of almost every meal. Drink at least three pints of water a day, and enjoy plenty of raw fruits and vegetables. Replace wine with fruit juice. Greatly reduce your intake of refined sugar, coffee, cola and tea. Enjoy apples, especially stewed

Case Study

Yvonne had suffered from a 'delicate' stomach since childhood. In addition, as she reached her early twenties, she developed bouts of sinusitis and catarrh that she could clear only with harsh coughing. Antibiotics were prescribed, but had little effect. As her symptoms became worse, Yvonne found them increasingly tiring, and embarrassing when she was with friends. Her sister suggested the problem could be an allergy to cows' milk and dairy products. In desperation, she began using soya milk with her morning cereal and eliminated dairy (cow's milk) products from all other food. The results were remarkable: 48 hours later the catarrh had almost cleared, and the pressure from her sinusitis was almost gone. To her surprise, she also found that she suffered fewer stomach cramps from gas. Her positive experience with this basic self-help process impressed her, and she wondered how much more improvement could be achieved with professional advice. She found a qualified nutrition therapist near her home, and sought help.

Yvonne was placed on a hypoallergenic diet, and told to eat less refined carbohydrate, and fewer foods made from grains. The list of foods she was advised to eat included zinc-rich fish, shellfish and seaweed, dark-green vegetables, fruit, and freshly ground pumpkin seeds, pulses and beans.

As Yvonne's health continued to improve, she realised that hers was a life-long problem of allergies that could be controlled by permanently altering her diet.

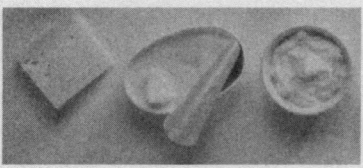

LEFT INTOLERANCES TO DAIRY PRODUCTS ARE VERY COMMON, AND MAY CAUSE SYMPTOMS INCLUDING CATARRH AND SINUS PROBLEMS.

apples, as dessert and in sauces with meat dishes. This condition is unpleasant in its own right, but also contributes to other conditions in the body.

CYSTITIS

Greatly increase your fluid intake to 2–3 litres (3–5 pints) a day. Part of this should be taken as cranberry juice, which is rich in a substance that prevents the bacteria that cause cystitis from sticking to the wall of your bladder. If they cannot stick, they will have no chance to multiply and cause infection.

DEPRESSION

Recent research has confirmed the important role that diet plays in controlling our moods. Low dietary levels of vitamin C, the B-complex vitamins and essential fatty acids should be corrected as a first step in treating depression. For the blues, try cutting down on alcohol and all caffeinated drinks, and increasing your consumption of wholegrains, soya, fresh fruits and green vegetables.

To avoid the 'sugar blues' (mood-swings caused by a sharp drop in your blood-sugar level), greatly reduce – or even eliminate – refined sugar from your diet.

If you are taking antidepressants, talk with your doctor about diet, but as a general rule avoid liver, alcohol, cheese, and canned and processed meats.

There are substances in chocolate that give a pleasant emotional state that has been described as similar to being in love. Some people use chocolate to aid depression for this reason, but

RIGHT CHOCOLATE MAY HAVE AN UPLIFTING EFFECT ON MOOD, BUT MAY CAUSE MIGRAINES IN SUSCEPTIBLE PEOPLE.

watch out for the side-effects of sugar (only eat chocolate with a cocoa content above 62%), and be aware that some people develop migraine headaches after eating chocolate.

DIARRHOEA

Eat grated apples and bananas to replace minerals, provide natural energy, and help clean the digestive system. Drink fruit juice and filtered water to replace lost fluid. Eat boiled rice and low-fibre food for 48 hours after the attack. Avoid spicy foods, coffee, tea, cola and alcohol for three or four days after the attack. Twenty-four hours after an attack, eat live yoghurt to help replenish normal gut flora. If you feel weak, add a pinch of table salt to a small glass of apple juice. Increase the proportion of antioxidant-rich red, orange and yellow fruits and vegetables in your diet. Wheatgerm and oatgerm added to food will help replace needed B-complex vitamins. If you suffer recurrent diarrhoea, include blueberries in your cooking. Like cranberries, they are a rich source of natural antibiotics.

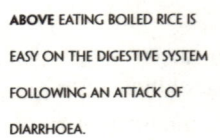

ABOVE EATING BOILED RICE IS EASY ON THE DIGESTIVE SYSTEM FOLLOWING AN ATTACK OF DIARRHOEA.

FATIGUE

Increase your intake of food high in complex carbohydrates, as these will help to stabilize your blood-sugar levels. Eliminate caffeinated drinks, alcohol and refined sugars from your diet. Eat foods rich in vitamin B12, zinc and folic acid (such as eggs, red meat, and dark green vegetables). Fatigue can be a symptom of many things. Consider consulting a nutritional therapist if you experience long-term fatigue.

Case Study

I recently had a student tell me she prepared a food diary, and realised how little complex carbohydrate she was eating. As a result, she began increasing her intake of bread, pasta and such foods. Within days, she was feeling less tired, and found she had enough energy to walk longer distances than she had in years. As a bonus, the exercise she enjoyed with her new-found energy resulted in firmer thighs and slimmer hips. Without knowing it, she had been denying her body the slow-releasing energy that she needed for normal well-being.

FLATULENCE

To avoid flatulence, try drinking mint or fennel tea and live yoghurt. Season your food with caraway, fennel seeds, thyme and sage. Caraway and fennel seeds can also be nibbled after eating foods that may produce gas. Foods that cause flatulence include cabbage, Brussel sprouts, and undercooked pulses.

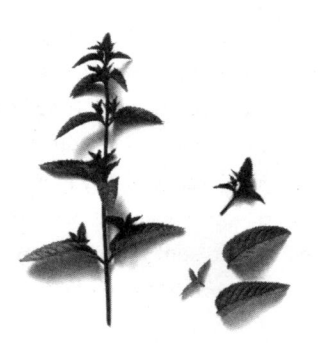

ABOVE MINT HAS A LONG HISTORY OF USE AS AN AID TO DIGESTION.

HALITOSIS (BAD BREATH)

This condition has many causes. To strengthen gums and fight gum disease, add raw apples to your diet and increase antioxidant levels by eating red and green fruits and vegetables. Greatly reduce your intake of sugar and sugary foods, as these lead to tooth decay and gum disease. The smell from infected sinuses can also cause bad breath. Select foods made with horseradish, mustard and ginger to help clear the condition.

NUTRITIONAL THERAPY

INDIGESTION AND HEARTBURN

Avoid all fried and fatty foods, caffeinated drinks – including colas – peppers, raw onions, and acid foods such as vinegar. Enjoy rice, wholegrain foods, and cooked vegetables. Try beer, or a drink made with Angostura bitters, about half an hour before a meal to stimulate the release of digestive juices. Also, eat slowly and chew your food well.

RIGHT IF YOU SUFFER FROM INDIGESTION AND HEARTBURN, TRY REDUCING YOUR INTAKE OF CAFFEINATED DRINKS SUCH AS COLAS, AS THEY ARE HIGHLY ACIDIC.

INFECTIONS

Chronic infections usually reflect a weakened immune system. Reduce your intake of refined sugar. Increase antioxidant-rich foods, such as red peppers and orange and yellow fruits and vegetables. Eat live yoghurt once a day. Eat oily fish twice a week or take fish oil supplements. Include soya products in your diet – including tofu, soya beans and soya yoghurt. Soya milk is an excellent drink. If skin lesions are present, you may wish to use supplements to increase your intake of zinc and vitamin C.

If you experience frequent infections, choose foods rich in antioxidants. Also add nuts to your food (unless you have an established nut allergy), and enjoy red and black fruits for dessert.

LEFT EATING SOYA PRODUCTS SUCH AS TOFU REGULARLY MAY HELP TO BUILD UP THE IMMUNE SYSTEM AND RESIST INFECTIONS.

SELF-HELP AND DISEASE PREVENTION

JOINT PAIN

Avoid obesity. Increase your intake of foods rich in selenium (nuts and cereals), vitamin C (fresh fruit and vegetables), vitamin E (nuts, avocados, virgin olive oil and sunflower seeds), and oily fish (for essential fatty acids). This combination of foods provides a balance of antioxidant vitamins and a good source of omega-3 fatty acids to help stimulate the presence of normal joint fluid.

ABOVE AVOCADOS ARE A GOOD SOURCE OF VITAMIN E, WHICH CAN HELP TO EASE JOINT PAIN.

MIGRAINE HEADACHES

Avoid alcohol (especially port and red wine), caffeine, cheese, citrus fruits and chocolate. Increase the amount of ginger in your cooking and drink fresh ginger tea. Increase your intake of oily fish. Eat regular meals; some people find that replacing three meals a day with five smaller meals is an effective way to control headaches.

LEFT RED WINE CAN TRIGGER MIGRAINE HEADACHES IN CERTAIN SUSCEPTIBLE PEOPLE.

MOUTH ULCERS

Recurrent mouth ulcers may be an indication of a compromised immune system. Try to boost your resistance by enjoying a healthy combination of foods rich in vitamin C, folic acid, B-vitamins, and zinc (nuts, fish, fruits and green vegetables and wholegrain foods). Avoid acid and salty foods.

OBESITY

Enjoy fish and lean meat, foods rich in complex carbohydrates (wholegrains, root vegetables and pulses), green salads and fresh fruit. Avoid refined sugar and cut down on all fats, especially animal fat. Reduce your total caloric intake. Eat raw and unprocessed foods. Processing removes nutrients from food and usually adds saturated fats and refined sugar.

OSTEOPOROSIS

This degenerative bone disease usually affects middle-aged and elderly women, but it can also affect men. Bones become brittle and easily fracture. The spine, ankle, wrists and hips are most vulnerable. Bone is a very active, living tissue, constantly being torn down and built up by two opposing groups of cells: the osteoclasts and osteoblasts. Oestrogen slows the action of cells that break down bone. Therefore, post-menopausal women are though to be particularly at risk.

Medical research has suggested that eating plenty of calcium-rich food during childhood and the teen years can minimize the risk of this potentially crippling disease. The diet for these groups should include plenty of dairy products and green leafy vegetables. Vitamin D should be provided either by exposure of the skin to sunlight, or via fortified foods, eggs and oily fish.

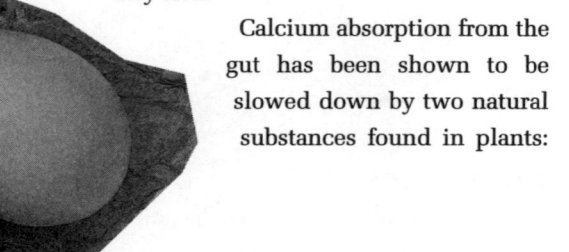

Calcium absorption from the gut has been shown to be slowed down by two natural substances found in plants:

LEFT EGGS ARE A GOOD SOURCE OF VITAMIN D, WHICH IS IMPORTANT IN THE PREVENTION OF OSTEOPOROSIS.

oxalic and phytic acids. Oxalic acid is found in rhubarb, spinach and chocolate; phytic acid is found in wheat bran, pulses and nuts. People concerned about osteoporosis should try to obtain most of the fibre they need from fruit and vegetables, and avoid foods containing phytic acid. Taking a daily supplement containing calcium and vitamin D has been shown to slow down bone loss.

High consumption of alcohol and caffeinated beverages is thought to encourage bone loss, and should therefore be reduced. Taking gentle exercise, however, strengthens bones and reduces mineral loss.

PREMENSTRUAL SYNDROME

Cut down your intake of salt, caffeine drinks and alcohol. Eat foods high in vitamin B6 (wholegrains, meat and fish), and linoleic acid (unrefined seed oils). This is a case where supplements have shown to be of great benefit. Use only the best quality evening primrose oil and vitamin B6.

RESTLESS LEGS

Restless legs can be an annoying problem, but one that is often overlooked as a health problem. The symptoms of the condition include 'pins and needles', a burning sensation in the legs, and involuntary muscle contractions and spasms. Stop smoking, lower your intake of salt and cut out caffeine.

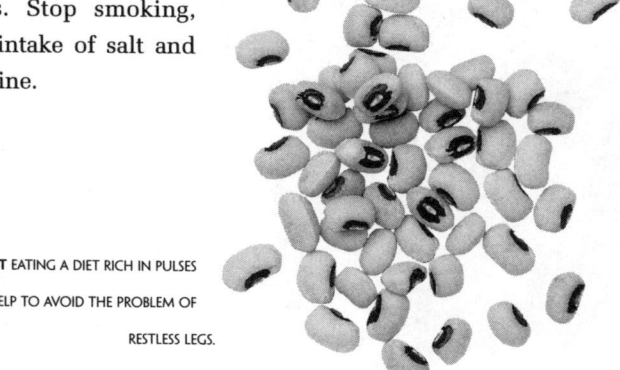

RIGHT EATING A DIET RICH IN PULSES CAN HELP TO AVOID THE PROBLEM OF RESTLESS LEGS.

Enjoy foods rich in vitamin B12, folic acid, iron, vitamin E and potassium (such as parsley, pulses, liver, unrefined oils, nuts, seeds and avocados).

STRESS

Stress is one of the most damaging factors of modern life. It contributes to the development of heart disease, cancer, the weakening of the immune system and emotional imbalance. Constant fatigue, depression, gastric upset, both constipation and diarrhoea, decreased sexual drive, lack of appetite, binge eating, muscle pain and memory loss can all result from stress. Stress distorts everything in your life, including the way you use your muscles, your posture, the way you sleep, and even the way you eat and digest your food. To manage stress in your life is to gain control over some of the most negative influences on both your health and appearance. Achieving control requires three things: relaxation, exercise and proper nutrition. Stress is worth an entire book to itself, but we only have room here to discuss how nutrition should fit into your stress-management plan.

Stress has many causes. Changes in the chemistry and physiology of the body, such as those caused by the menstrual cycle, add to the demand for all the B vitamins, although B6 appears to play a special role in reducing symptoms.

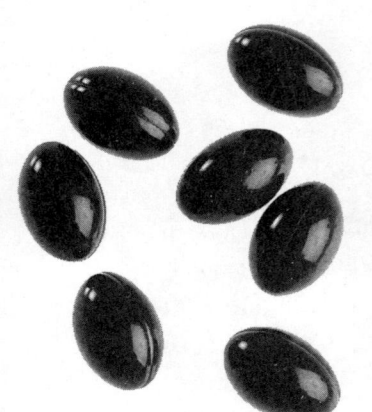

Key micronutrients involved in combating stress include B vitamins, vitamin C and zinc. All the nutrients grouped as B-complex vitamins are essential for normal brain and nerve function. These are thiamin (B1), riboflavin (B2), niacin (B3), pantothenic acid (B5), pyridoxine (B6), cobalamin

LEFT SUPPLEMENTS SUCH AS ZINC MAY HELP THE BODY TO DEAL WITH THE EFFECTS OF STRESS.

(B12), folic acid and biotin. As these are all water-soluble vitamins, they are not stored in the body, and a fresh supply must be made available each day. Vitamin C is also water-soluble, and stress increases the use and therefore demand for this vital nutrient. As the immune system is weakened by stress, the mineral zinc is essential for maintaining optimum physical and mental performance when you are under pressure. Remember that zinc works in conjunction with magnesium, another essential mineral, which is rapidly excreted from the body. Under stressful conditions, the body uses these nutrients with speed, and quantities larger than normal may be required for the smooth functioning of the brain and nerves.

Eat small, frequent meals containing good sources of complex carbohydrates to help sustain a near-constant blood-sugar level rather than the energy rushes and slumps with eating refined sugars. Chew food well and slowly, incorporating your mouth enzymes to help break down your food. Reduce – or better still – eliminate alcoholic beverages. Finally, avoid caffeinated drinks – coffee, cola, tea, chocolate, and drink teas that relax your mind and body; both camomile and passionflower teas are highly recommended. Avoid over-processed and refined foods, and eat organic foods whenever possible. Add oatgerm or wheatgerm to your food, and enjoy freshly ground seeds and nut butters. Try skipping alcohol for a few days and see if you feel better. St. John's wort, a herbal remedy, helps to take the edge off stress in many people. Stress may also be helped by a hypoallergenic diet (see Chapter 5).

VAGINITIS

Eat a portion of live yoghurt daily. Enjoy four or five small meals instead of three larger ones; include a good source of protein with each. Add seeds, nuts, wheatgerm and oatgerm to your food. Increase your intake of vegetables and pulses, especially foods high in antioxidant vitamins. Avoid refined sweets and eat limited quantities of dried fruit.

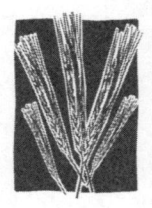

FOOD AND BEAUTY

CHAPTER NINE

Beauty consists of more than fine features and a firm body. It is an inner glow, a look of contentment, and the gleam of fresh skin and healthy hair. Without these, the fine features and firm body are dull and lifeless. With these, a person with ordinary features and an ordinary body can be beautiful.

Balanced nutrition is vital to beauty, and although this book deals primarily with food and illness, the subject of appearance should not be overlooked. Three important aspects of beauty covered here are hair, nails and skin.

HAIR

The condition of your hair reflects your general level of well-being. Illness, stress, and inadequate levels of important nutrients cause changes in the parts of the scalp that produce and protect each strand of hair. These changes take time to put right. While it is true that harsh treatment and too much sun also destroy the lustre and strength of hair, nutritional deficiencies are the hair's worst enemy.

DRY HAIR AND DANDRUFF

These may be caused by a zinc deficiency. Eat more pumpkin seeds, shellfish and red meat. Increase your intake of foods rich in essential fatty acids. Increase the number of antioxidant-rich foods in your diet. Cut down on alcoholic beverages and salt. You may be suffering from a food allergy, and should consider a hypoallergenic diet. Try eliminating citrus fruit, wheat and dairy products.

HAIR LOSS

This is common in men, and can be caused by a number of conditions in women, including thyroid disease, anaemia and pregnancy. If you have symptoms of these conditions, seek medical advice. Pregnancy may also change the condition of your hair if you do not eat a well-balanced diet. In general, increase your intake of colourful foods, such as dried apricots, carrots, red sweet peppers and green leafy vegetables to provide the beta-carotene your body needs to make vitamin A. Eat two or three eggs a week, and – unless you are pregnant – eat liver once a week.

Stress can also cause hair loss. Increase your intake of B-vitamins if you think this could be a problem. Heavy metal poisoning may cause hair loss, and a detoxifying diet may help. Crash dieting, mono-diets and yo-yo dieting can also damage your hair and cause loss.

GREASY HAIR

In addition to frequent washing with a good shampoo, try reducing the quantity of refined sugar you eat. Protein is the major substance in hair, so make certain your diet includes enough of this important macronutrient.

NAILS

The condition of your nails conveys much about your health. If they are very pale and brittle, you may be anaemic and need more iron in your diet. If the thumbnails are spoon-shaped, and turn up, you may be low on both zinc and iron. Zinc deficiency can also show up as white spots on the nails, although these most often are from a knock or hard bump.

Too much of the mineral selenium will cause black nails, whereas too little in the diet causes wide bands or ridges on the nails.

Blueish nails indicate poor circulation, and the condition should be checked by a health practitioner.

For healthy nails, follow the advice as for healthy hair. Note, however, that it is not true that calcium supplements will build strong nails. One tip – the tannin in tea disrupts the absorption of iron into the body, and may contribute to anaemia.

SKIN

I was once told by a dermatologist that she chose that speciality because the skin is like a road-map showing a person's past life: clues to every major illness, what they ate and how they lived could be found if one knew where to look. Covering the body to stop us from losing water and protecting us against the invasion of foreign organisms, regulating the body's temperature through sweating and the flexing of tiny hairs, the skin is far more complex than we often imagine.

The nutrients needed for healthy skin include: zinc, vitamins A, C, and biotin (a member of the B-complex) and essential fatty acids. A well-balanced diet that supports healthy skin should include red, green, yellow and orange fruits and vegetables; nuts pulses and shellfish; eggs, wheatgerm and vegetable oils.

Other tips for healthy skin: abnormal levels of free radicals damage the delicate structures in the skin, and should be avoided when possible. Do not smoke, and restrict your exposure to the sun. Include as many antioxidant-rich foods in your diet as possible. Enjoy one or two good-sized portions of protein-rich food each day, but restrict your intake of red meat. Saturated animal fats should be avoided. Add nuts, seeds and sprouts – especially alfalfa sprouts – to salads, sandwiches and use to garnish other dishes. Drink plenty of water. Cut down on tea, coffee and alcohol. Supplement your diet with

Evening Primrose Oil or other compounds rich in gamma-linoleic acid [GLA]. Try avoiding cheese and foods containing chocolate: a link may exist between eczema and intolerance to these foods.

If you suffer from acne, boost your vitamin C intake by increasing the amount of fresh fruit and vegetables that you eat. Improve your level of dietary zinc by adding more lean meat, poultry, shellfish and nuts to your diet. Reduce your intake of sweet and salty treats.

ABOVE EATING PLENTY OF FRESH FRUIT AND VEGETABLES WILL HELP TO IMPROVE YOUR SKIN.

SMOKING AND WRINKLES

An important beauty tip: if you want to avoid wrinkles, do not smoke. If you smoke – stop. Many young women are smoking these days, and they will deeply regret this habit in years to come. We have known for decades that smoking increases the risk of deadly illnesses; apply that knowledge to your own life, and enjoy a better life longer.

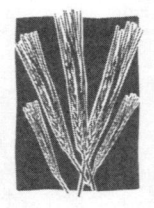

CONSULTING A NUTRITIONAL THERAPIST

CHAPTER TEN

Having learnt something about the power of nutritional healing, you may want to seek advice from an expert who can use their knowledge of nutrition to help you solve your health problems.

PREPARING FOR A CONSULTATION

There are certain things that you may find it helpful to do before consulting a nutritional therapist.
- Consider your budget. Help from an expert has a price. But keep in mind that a short period of help from a qualified person can be highly effective.
- Identify specific symptoms or changes in your body that concern you. For example, a marked whitening of your finger nails, bouts of indigestion after meals, arthritic joint pain, and so on. Think carefully about changes in your body and write them down.
- Ask yourself if you are prepared to change your eating habits. Giving up enjoyable foods is difficult, even when you know they are causing health problems. Before seeking help, decide to follow the advice given.

- Consider whether you will need help fitting your new diet into the usual pattern of family meals. Enlist the support of your family and friends even before you talk to an expert. Make people understand that you are making an important change in your lifestyle.

FINDING A THERAPIST

Just a decade ago, it was difficult to find well-trained nutrition therapists in large cities, and almost impossible to find one in a rural area. Happily, as interest in nutrition has grown, things have changed. Now there are national organisations to contact and ask for the names and addresses of experts near you. (See Useful Addresses.) While making enquiries, request information about the organisations you contact: what qualifications are required for membership, are the standards of care set by the group, how complaints are dealt with, and so on. It may be tempting to thumb through the telephone directory looking for the name of a nutritional therapist with a local address, but remember – if after seeking help you later have a complaint, or questions about your therapist's practice, you will have no professional body to contact for guidance.

Once you have identified a nutritionist, contact them requesting information about the nature of the service they provide, and about their training and experience. Wait to receive some form of response, such as a brochure, before taking the proceedings any further. Some therapists will work with you over the telephone; others will not begin treatment until they have talked with you extensively in person. Many nutritionists will require you to give blood and urine samples for them to analyze before they prescribe specific dietary changes or the use of supplements. Others may use hair samples to gain information about your general health status.

What to Expect

As a first step, you will have a chance to describe the problems for which you are seeking help. Do not withhold facts about the causes of stress in your life, or physical symptoms that may be embarrassing to talk about. If your digestive pain is accompanied by passing gas – say so. If you leak urine every time you cough – report that. Also, be honest about your food intake: do not underestimate the numbers of bouts of compulsive eating you have experienced during the past month. If there are foods that you strongly dislike – say so. If there are cultural or family problems that may make it difficult for you to change your eating patterns, explain that to the therapist. The more complete the information you give the therapist, the better the help he or she can give you.

The nutritionist will ask questions about your lifestyle, dietary habits, family medical history, and general physical health. You will probably be asked to keep a food diary for a certain amount of time. To gain understanding of what is happening in your body, blood, urine and hair samples may be requested.

After your assessment, the nutritional therapist will review your case and recommend dietary changes. These may be simple - cutting down on refined sugar, for instance – or extensive. For example, if the results show that you are allergic to gluten, you may need to make many modifications in your food choices. But do not worry about this; your therapist will help you to identify appropriate alternatives, and even suggest retail sources for these items.

Supplements may also be added to your health regime. Follow instructions prescribed for you, and report any changes in the way you feel – both positive and negative – to your therapist. You may find your body requires a large number of supplements at the beginning of your treatment, but your regime will be simplified as your health improves.

There may be times when the positive effect of supplements will go beyond those you anticipate. For example, Evening Primrose Oil

[EPO], frequently used to control premenstrual syndrome, can also greatly improve the condition of your nails and hair.

Keep in mind that nutritional therapy may not alter symptoms as quickly as pharmaceutical drugs. Sometime the effects are immediate: I have seen cases of milk allergy where a longstanding case of lung congestion, phlegm and coughing is improved within 48 hours simply by totally eliminating cows' milk from the diet. Other treatments may take weeks or months before the full effects are enjoyed. As an example, improving skin conditions requires a rebuilding of tissue cells, which takes time. If the improvements you seek are slow in coming, do not give up. Discuss the situation with your therapist. Remember that cheating on your diet or supplements slows things down.

If your nutritional therapist spots symptoms of a condition requiring medical intervention – diabetes or cancer for example - she or he will tell you. Under these circumstances, working with your GP and nutritionist together can be very effective, providing that both agree on the action to take.

Case Study

Alan, an accountant, suffered an outbreak of cold sores on his lower lip every time the level of stress built up at work. This was not only uncomfortable, but also unsightly and embarrassing when working with clients. He sought help from his doctor, but the medicated cream prescribed was only moderately effective. Concerned, Alan's boss suggested that he consult a nutritional therapist for advice. After carefully reviewing his history of physical complaints and eating habits, the nutritionist explained that Alan needed to strengthen his immune system. She suggested he avoid alcohol, animal fat, refined sugar and all caffeinated drinks, and prescribed a diet avoiding citrus fruit and all foods rich in arginine (an amino acid building-block of protein found in almonds, peanuts, chicken and wheat). She also told him to increase the amount of garlic and onions that he ate, use vegetable oils as a source of vitamin E, and increase his intake of fruits and vegetables rich in the antioxidant vitamins A and C.

To restore and build up the nutrient base needed to support his immune system, Alan was placed on a three-month course of food supplements containing antioxidants vitamins A and C and the mineral selenium. He was also advised to take supplements containing L-lysine (an amino acid that helps inhibit the reproduction of viruses), take echinacea – a plant thought to be rich in natural antibiotics, and drink a daily dose of Aloe vera juice.

After a few weeks, Alan generally felt better, but had no proof that his therapist's advice was working until, six months later, a crisis occurred with one of his clients. He sailed through events with no sign of a distressing outbreak of cold sores. Soon after, his nutritional therapist discharged him, with instructions to maintain a careful watch on what he ate.

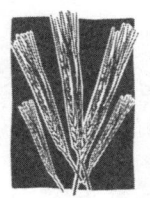

TAKING IT FURTHER

CHAPTER ELEVEN

Nutrition is arguably the most exciting and rapidly developing of the healing arts. It combines the latest medical research with the most fundamental and ancient knowledge of the human body. It is an aid to both the body and the mind. It directly links your body and its functions with the very stuff of life: the nutrients. Medical research proves the links between poor diet and disease, and the demand for trained nutritionists has greatly increased. For those who enjoy working with people, and have considered entering a helping profession, training as a nutritional therapist may be a good career choice.

Many qualified nutritional therapists establish their own clinics, and practise independently. Others work in teams, or with members of other healing professions in surgeries, clinics and hospitals. Many medical doctors are training in nutritional therapy. This is a great step forward, opening the door to better care for patients and for greater co-operation between traditional medicine and nutritional therapy.

Training varies widely and in some countries there are few regulations governing the qualifications a therapist needs to practise. However, as more nutritionists set up clinics and treat people with serious problems, stricter rules regulating the training needed by practitioners are sure to follow. Remember: if you decide to become a nutritional therapist, be sure to ask how various training programmes will qualify you for certification in the future. This is important to keep in mind from the beginning, because it could greatly influence the type of practice and the fees you will be able to charge.

Training programmes vary in length and design. Some are a few weeks long, others take years. Some are based in colleges and universities, and others are run by independent organisations. The best programmes offer opportunities for continuing education, so consider that as you investigate your options. In some places you need not have a university degree before training as a nutritional therapist, and you can combine the study of nutrition with other healing arts.

If you are scientifically minded, you may wish to participate in the investigative aspect of nutrition. If you are already trained in a science discipline, you may only need to find the right employer. However, if your scientific background is limited, local universities are good places to begin your search for training. You may even wish to pursue a research degree programme leading to a doctorate. Again, training varies according to your interests, and may take place in university departments as seemingly diverse as Food Technology and Biochemistry. Alternatively, if you want to treat patients, but in a research setting rather than in the community, you could consider training as a medical doctor and adding a degree in nutrition later.

Always remember that no matter what form of nutrition training you choose — you can always add to your understanding and practice through subsequent training in another field of holistic or alternative medicine.

If you think you would find a rewarding career in nutrition, first consider the following:
- Do you enjoy working with people?
- Do you enjoy learning and updating yourself on medical and scientific subjects?
- Do you like or dislike the feeling of responsibility that comes with giving advice that you know will affect another person's well-being?

- What financial rewards are you seeking?
- Would you want to work from home, or in a clinic or institutional setting?
- How much effort are you willing to put into your training?
- How much can you afford to spend on training? Do you have access to funds, or know of sources for funds to cover your living expenses while you train?

After considering these issues, you may want to talk with someone currently practising as a nutritional therapist. If you need a contact, look in the telephone directory for a list of practitioners near you. Write and ask several if you can talk with them about your career interests and their professional experiences. It is always surprising how much time people are willing to give if they think you are sincerely interested. When you have such an opportunity, plan what you want to ask before the interview, keep to any agreed schedule for the interview, and make certain the person you talk with understands how much you appreciate their help. The kinds of questions you will want to ask include: where they trained, what that training was like, what educational credentials they had before training, and what professional credentials they gained.

Glossary

Amino acid: The smallest building block of protein. The human body cannot manufacture eight of the twenty amino acids that it contains. These eight (sometimes nine) amino acids are called 'essential' amino acids, and must be obtained from food.

Antibodies: Powerful molecules produced by the immune system that specifically attack and destroy invading viruses and bacteria. This is the main line of defence against infection. In some illnesses antibodies are produced that attack and damage the normal tissues of the body.

Anticarcinogens: Compounds found in plants that are thought to prevent, destroy or reduce the growth of cancer cells. Food from cruciferous plants, including broccoli, cabbage, Brussels sprouts, kale and mustard leaves are sources of one type of anticarcinogens. Others are found in soya, onions and garlic.

Antioxidant: Molecules that counter the damaging reactive nature of free radicals.

Antiviral compounds: Certain foods, such as garlic, contain compounds thought to destroy viruses or prevent their duplication.

Autoimmune disease: a condition produced when the body develops an allergy to one or more of its own tissues.

Bioflavonoids: Powerful natural antioxidants that work with vitamin C to strengthen the smallest blood vessels, called capillaries; they are also thought to help prevent certain forms of cancer.

Calories: The basic unit to describe a specific amount of energy. A calorie (c) is very small, making it inappropriate for use when describing energy in food. Kilocalories (Kcal) or Calories (C) both represent 1000 calories, and are used when calculating diets and human energy needs.

Catabolism: The processes by which the body breaks down substances from food.

Co-enzymes: Compounds in foods that speed up the action of enzymes. Co-enzymes may be vitamins, minerals, or other compounds produced by the body. When the body fails to obtain adequate levels of co-enzymes from the diet, or fails to produce enough on its own, important biochemical processes in the body can fail to function.

DNA (Deoxyribonucleic acid): The blueprint of the human body found in all cells. It carries the genetic code that determines all biochemical processes.

Enzymes: Protein compounds produced by the body that speed up natural biochemical processes without being used themselves.

EPO: Evening Primrose Oil; a rich source of GLA (gamma-linolenic acid), an essential omega-6 fatty acid needed for normal tissue health and regulation.

Fatty acid: The smallest building block of a simple fat (triglyceride). Certain fatty acids are essential for normal growth and tissue function. Depending on their molecular structure, essential fatty acids are classified as either omega-3 or omega-6. Both are necessary for normal cell structures and as parts of small messenger molecules in the body. EPA and DHA are common names for omega-3 essential fatty acids, found in oily fish. GLA is an essential omega-6 fatty acid found in seed oils from plants, including starflower (also known as borage) and evening primrose.

Fibre: The indigestible parts of food from plants. Soluble fibre, as found in oats, is thought to help reduce blood cholesterol levels. Insoluble fibre provides the bulk needed to clear the lower digestive tract.

Free radical: A highly reactive molecule that occurs in the body and can disrupt and damage other molecules in its environment.

Hormones: Messenger molecules produced by various parts of the body that travel through the blood stream and affect organs and tissues elsewhere.

Malabsorption: Failure by the digestive system to absorb nutrients from the intestinal tract.

ME (Myalgic Encephalitis, also known as **Chronic Fatigue**

Syndrome): A continuing state of exhaustion, thought to follow some viral infections, which is made worse by a poor balance of essential nutrients.

Metabolism: Chemical processes in the body that break down the food we eat and build up the molecules and structures of the body.

Microgram: 1000th of a milligram.

Milligram: 1000th of a gram.

Minerals: Inorganic substances used in the normal biological processes of life.

Nutrients: Constituents of food and drink essential for health.

Nutrition: The balance between the demand for, and availability of, the necessary constituents of food. Optimal nutrition is the ideal balance of all nutrients. Super nutrition is a balance of nutrients that tips in favour of oversupply of certain protective nutrients.

Oestrogen: A hormone that controls female sexual development.

Oxidation: Chemical processes involving the combining of oxygen with other compounds.

Phytochemicals: Natural compounds in plants that are biologically active in the human body, but play no essential part in the basic biological processes in human cells.

Phytoestrogens: Substances in plants that are similar in form to the oestrogen found in women. They are thought to reduce the physical symptoms of oestrogen depletion, and protect against certain forms of oestrogen-dependent cancers.

Prostaglandins: A large group of molecules produced in the body and incorporating essential fatty acids. They act as regulators of blood flow, nerve activity, hormonal activity, gastrointestinal function and other biological functions.

Starch: Complex carboydrates that are the greatest store of energy available to the body from food.

Vitamins: natural substances that the human body cannot make for itself, but are essential parts of vital chemical processes in the body.

FURTHER READING

Balancing Hormones Naturally, Kate Neil and Patrick Holford, Piatkus, London, 1998

A Barefoot Doctor's Manual, prepared by The Revolutionary Health Committee of Hunan Province, Routledge & Kegan Paul, London and Henley, 1978

The Better Pregnancy Diet, Patrick Holford and Liz Lorente, ION Press, London 1992

The Book of Green Tea, by Diana Rosen, Storey Books, 1998

The Estrogen Decision, Susan Lark, M.D., Celestial Arts, USA, 1995

The Everyday Wheat-Free Gluten-Free Cookbook, Michelle Berriedale-Johnson, Grub Street, London, 1999

The Fats We Need to Eat, Jeannette Ewin Ph. D., Thorsons/HarperCollins, London, 1995

Food and Cancer Prevention: Chemical and Biological Aspects, edited by K.W. Waldron, I.T. Johnson and G.R. Fenwick, The Royal Society of Chemistry, Cambridge, England, 1993

The Food Pharmacy, Jean Carper, Simon & Schuster, London, 1989,

The Green Pharmacy, James A. Duke, Rodale Press, Emmaus, Pennsylvania, USA, 1997

Healing Through Nutrition, Dr. Melvyn R. Werbach, HarperCollins, 1995

Healing with Whole Foods: Oriental Traditions and Modern Medicine, Paul Pitchford, Revised Edition, North Atlantic Books, California, 1993

Health Essentials: Vitamin Guide, Hasnain Walji, Element Books, United Kingdom, 1992

A Life in Balance: The Complete guide to Ayurvedic Nutrition and Body Types with Recipes, Maya Tiwari, Healing Arts Press, Vermont, USA, 1995

Manual of Natural Family Planning, Dr Anna M. Flynne and Melissa Brooks, Thorsons, London, 1996

Miracle Cures, Jean Carper, (BCA) HarperCollins Publishers, 1997

Native Nutrition: Eating according to ancestral wisdom, Ronald F. Schmid, Healing Arts Press, Vermont, USA, 1987

Natural Alternatives to HRT, Dr Marilyn Glenville, Kyle Cathie Limited, London, 1997

Natural Alternatives to Over-the-Counter and Prescription Drugs, Michael T Murray, William Morrow, New York, 1994

No More PMS, Maryon and Dr Alan Stewart, Vermilion, London, 1997

Nutrition and Evolution, Michael Crawford and David Marsh, Airlift, 1995

Nutritional Healing, Denise Mortimore, Element Books, United Kingdom, 1998

Nutritional Medicine, Dr Stephen Davies & Dr Alan Stewart, Pan Books, London, 1987

The Osteoporosis Solution, Carl Germano, RD, CNS, LDN, and William Cabot M.D., Kensington Books, New York, 1999

The Plants we Need to Eat, Jeannette Ewin, Ph.D. Thorsons/HarperCollins, London, 1997

Professional Products Manual, Quest International, Birmingham, UK, 1997

Useful Addresses

CANADA
National Institute of Nutrition
2565 Carling Avenue, Suite 400
Ottawa, Ontario
K 8RI

NEW ZEALAND
New Zealand Natural
Health Practitioners
Accreditation
Board
P.O. Box 37–491
Auckland

UNITED KINGDOM
Ayurvedic Medical
Association UK
The Hale Clinic
7 Park Crescent
London
W1N 3HE
020 7631 0156 (your
message will be
passed on)

B.A.N.T. (British
Association of
Nutritional Therapists)
BCM – B.A.N.T
London
WC1N 3XX
0870 606 1284

Bristol Cancer Help Centre
Grove House
Cornwallis Grove
Clifton
Bristol BS8 4PG
0117 980 9500
www.bristolcancerhelp.org

British Society for Allergy,
Environmental and
Nutritional Medicine
P.O. Box 7
Knighton
LD7 1WT
Information line: 0906 302 0010
Books and other printed
materials: 01703 812124
A society of physicians
who recognise the broad
benefits of nutritional
healing. A list of members
is available from
the information line.

Institute for Optimum Nutrition
Blades Court,
Deodar Road
London SW15 2NU
General information:
020 8877 9993
Fax: 020 8877 9980
e-mail: info@ion.ac.uk

National Institute of Medical
Herbalists
56 Longbrook Street
Exeter
Devon
EX4 6AH
01392 426022
nimh@ukexeter.freeserve.co.uk

Nutrition Society
10 Cambridge Court
210 Shepherd's Bush Road
London
W6 7NJ
020 7602 0228
www.nutsoc.org.uk

Register of Chinese Herbal
Medicine
P.O.Box 400
Wembley
Middlesex
HA9 9NZ
07000 790332
www.rchm.co.uk

Institute of Complementary
Medicine
P.O.Box 194
London
SE16 7QZ
(British register of
complementary practitioners)
020 7237 5165

Society for the Promotion of
Nutritional Therapy (S.P.N.T)
St Albans
Hertfordshire
AL3 7ZQ
01582 792 088
Registration body for nutritional therapists. Publishes Nutritional Therapy Today, a journal for members. For more information on nutritional therapy and a list of practitioners, send £1.00 and a S.A.E to the above address.

The Nutri Centre
7 Park Crescent
London
W1N 3HE
www.nutricentre.com
Supplements, books
and reference:
020 7323 2382
The Nutri Centre is a naturopathic dispensary that also provides a reference library, bookshop and mail order service.

The Soil Association
Bristol House
40-56 Victoria Street
Bristol, BS1 6BY
0117 929 0661
www.soilassociation.org

Higher Nature
The Nutrition Centre
Burwash Common
East Sussex
TN19 7LX
Direct line for nutritional
advice: 01435 882964
Business number: 01435 883484
www.highernature.co.uk

Nature's Best Health Products
Century Place
Tunbridge Wells
Kent
TN2 3BE
Nutrition advice line:
01892 534143

Quest Vitamins Ltd
Nutrition Department
8 Venture Way
Aston Science Park
Birmingham
B7 4AP
0121 359 0056
Fax: 0121 359 0313
e-mail:
info@questvitamins.co.uk
www.questvitamins.co.uk

Solgar
(nutritionists available at large chemists, such as John Bell and Croyden in London)

The Marketing Department
Solgar Vitamins Ltd
Beggars Lane
Aldbury
Tring
Hertfordshire
HP23 5PT
For more information on local suppliers: 01442 890355
www.solgar.com

UNITED STATES
OF AMERICA
American College of Alternative Medicine
P.O. Box 3427
Laguna Hills
CA 92654

American Dietetic Association
216 W. Jackson Blvd.
Suite 800
Chicago
IL 60606

American Association for Health Freedom
9912 Georgetown Pike
Suite D-2, P.O. Box 458
Great Falls
VA 22066
800 230 2762
www.apma.net

COURSES
UNITED KINGDOM
Foundation for Applied
Nutrition
133 Gately Road
Gately, Cheadle
Cheshire SK8 4PD

Institute for Optimum Nutrition
(ION)
5 Jerdan Place
London
SW6 1BE

Woman to Woman
PO Box 2252
Brighton
East Sussex
BN3 6BU

SOUTH AFRICA
Natural Health Association
PO BOX 39556
Bramley
2018

Natural Health Clinic
Complementary Therapies
PO BOX 6299
Halfway House
1685

INDEX

ageing 22–3
alfalfa sprouts 66
algae 66
allergies 36–7, 94
allium 66
aloe vera 67
amino acids 29, 45–6, 50–1, 87
anaemia 82
anatomy 25
anise 67
anti-cancer foods 72–3
anti-Candida diets 38–9
antioxidants 62–4, 92
ascorbic acid 12–13, 55–6
Ayurvedic healing 8–9

balanced diet 7, 17
Barefoot Doctors 10–11
beauty 104–7
blueberries 67
body
  changes 20
  harmony 25
  types 8–9
boron 59

caffeine 37
calcium 58
calories 31, 85
cancer 72–3, 90–3
candidiasis 93
carbohydrates 32, 49, 97
cardiovascular disease 89–90
carrots 67
catarrh 93
chewing 42
childhood 20
Chinese medicine 10–11
cholesterol 53
chromium 59
cold sores 111–12
constipation 93–5
consultations 108
copper 59–60
cranberries 67
Cruciferous plant family 93
cystitis 95

dandruff 104–5
deficiencies 32–3
depression 95
detoxification 33
diarrhoea 96
diets
  ageing 22–3
  anti-Candida 38–9
  balanced 7, 17
  elimination 37
  Hay 34
  high-protein 31
  hypoallergenic 34–6, 94
  illness 23–4
  menopause 22
  mono-diets 38
  pregnancy 21
  vegan 29
  weight-loss 30–1
digestive system 40–4
dill 68
disease prevention 14–15, 83
doshas 8–9
dry hair 104–5

eating habits 30
edible plants 65–73
education 113–15

elimination diets 37
Evening Primrose oil 107, 110–11
exercise 17, 85
exhaustion 81–2

factory analogy 25–6
fasting 38
fat consumption 27, 85
fatigue 96
fats 52–3
fennel 68
fibre 49–50, 91
finding a therapist 109
fingernails 105–6
flatulence 97
food
  combinations 29, 34
  diary 110
  supplements 74
  types 48
free radicals 62–3, 106

grapes 68
greasy hair 105
green tea 69

hair 104–5
halitosis 97
Hay diet 34
headaches 36, 99
health 7, 18–19
heart disease 89–90
herbs 73
high-protein diets 31
Hippocrates 11
holistic healing 8
hypoallergenic diets 34–6, 94

illness
  diets 23–4
  digestive 40–1
  free radicals 63
  nutritional deficiencies 86
  physical 18–19
immune system 87–8, 111–12
indigestion 98
infections 98
insoluble fibre 50
intestines 43
iodine 60
iron 60

joint pain 99
juicing 38

lemons 13

lifestyle 16, 110
Lind, James 12–13
liver function 44
loss of hair 105

macrominerals 58–9
macronutrients 49
magnesium 58
malnutrition 16
man-made chemicals 83–4
manganese 60–1
manufacturers, supplements 76
meat, amino acids 51
menopause 22
metabolism 44–6
micronutrients 53
migraines 36, 99
milk allergies 36
minerals 33, 57–8, 75
moderation 46
molybdenum 61
mono-diets 38
mouth ulcers 99

nightshade plant family 35

INDEX

non-food plants 71–2
nutrients 47–8, 75
nutritional supplements 28, 74–82, 110–11

obesity 100
olive oil 69
organic foods 24
osteoporosis 100
overdosing, supplements 76–7

parsley 69
phosphorus 59
physical illness 18–19
phytochemicals 27, 92
pineapple 70
plant remedies 65
potassium 61
pre-menstrual syndrome (PMS) 101
pre-menstrual tension (PMT) 80–1
pregnancy 21
processed food 84–5
protein 45–6, 50

qualifications 113–15

Recommended Daily Allowances (RDAs) 14–15
recovery, speed of 111
research 15–16, 113
restless legs 101

safety levels, supplements 79–80
scurvy 12
selenium 61–2
skin problems 106–7
smoking 91, 107
snacks 32
sodium 59
solanine 35
soluble fibre 50
soya beans 70
spices 9, 73
stomach 42–3
stress 102–3
sunlight, skin 106
supplements 28, 74–82, 110–11
symptoms, analyzing 110
therapists, nutritional 108–12
thyroid gland 44–5
tinctures 71
tomatoes 69
toxins 27–8, 33, 57
trace minerals 59–62
training 113–15

university degrees 114

vaginitis 103
vegan diets 29, 87
vitamins
  A–E 53–7
  antioxidants 63–4
  C 12–13, 55–6
  supplements 75

waste products 43–4
water 24, 49
weight-loss 30–1
well-being 17–19

yams 70
Yin and Yang 10
youth 18

127